CLINICAL INVESTIGATION AND STATISTICS IN LABORATORY MEDICINE

'A statistical analysis, properly conducted, is a delicate dissection of uncertainties, a surgery of suppositions. The surgeon must guard carefully against false incisions with his scalpel. Very often he has to sew the patient up as inoperable.'

M J Moroney
Facts from Figures

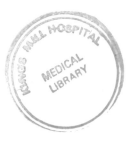
MANAGEMENT AND TECHNOLOGY IN
LABORATORY MEDICINE

Series Editors: Gwyn McCreanor BSc, MSc, PhD, MRCPath
Roy A Sherwood BSc, MSc, DPhil
Guest Editors: Sally Hollis BSc, MSc and R Andrew Moore MA, DPhil, CChem, FRSC

CLINIC. ...~~~INVESTIGATION~~ AND STATISTICS
IN LABORATORY MEDICINE

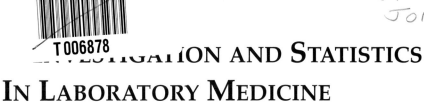

Richard G Jones, MRCP
Senior Lecturer in Chemical Pathology, University of Leeds
and Honorary Consultant Chemical Pathologist, Institute of Pathology,
United Leeds Teaching Hospitals Trust.

R Brian Payne, MD, PhD, FRCPath
Formerly Consultant Chemical Pathologist, St James's University Hospital
and Senior Clinical Lecturer in Chemical Pathology, University of Leeds.

A C B VENTURE PUBLICATIONS

ACB VENTURE PUBLICATIONS
Chairman and Managing Editor - David Burnett

MANAGEMENT AND TECHNOLOGY IN LABORATORY MEDICINE
Series Editors - Gwyn McCreanor and Roy A Sherwood

British Library Cataloguing in Publication Data

A catalogue record for the book is available from the British Library

ISBN 0 902429 21 3 ACB Venture Publications

Cover Design - Mike Webb of M J Webb Associates

Cover Plate taken from The Life, Letters and Labours of Francis Galton by Karl Pearson showing the Quincunx used to demonstrate the laws of natural selection

Printed by Piggott Printers (Cambridge) Ltd

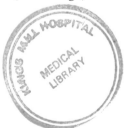

Preface

This book is designed for people working in clinical and laboratory medicine who "don't know enough statistics" and who develop a mental block when faced with a text filled with equations. It should help them to design investigations and to analyse their data using a problem-solving approach. We have made liberal use of diagrams and illustrations but very sparing use of equations and symbols. (It has been said that there are more symbols needed in statistics than there are letters in the Greek and Roman alphabets!) The book is not intended to be read like an automobile engineer's manual, explaining in detail how statistical methods work; but to be more like a road map, an itinerary and a Highway Code, making it simple to travel from the starting point, definition of the question, through collection and validation of data and its analysis using the best statistical program to the destination, interpretation of the results.

The book is organised into four main Chapters. The first describes the different kinds of data and the statistical analyses that can be applied to them. The second deals with the inaccuracy, imprecision, detection limit and other aspects of analytical methods used in laboratory medicine. The third describes how to obtain and use data for diagnosis and for monitoring patients. The final Chapter, the design of clinical experiments, requires a knowledge of the other Chapters but is a good starting point for clinical investigation.

We have assumed that the reader will have access to a computer with statistical software for inspection and analysis of data. The statistical package we recommend, Analyse-IT (Smart Software) functions as an integral part of Microsoft Excel. Among the programs provided are three ways of generating descriptive statistics depending on whether the data are analysed as single, multiple or sequenced data sets; a range of transform functions; sample size calculators; and seventeen commonly used parametric and non-parametric statistical tests with graphical displays and confidence intervals where appropriate. Analyse-IT features ten statistical programs not readily available elsewhere that are of particular interest to those who work in clinical and laboratory medicine. The programs include tests for the Normality of a distribution, both Deming regression and Passing/Bablok regression, Altman and Bland method comparison and both Galen and Gambino and ROC analysis.

We have added a little human interest: brief biographies of five scientists who made major contributions to the development of medical statistics and evidence-based medicine - Gauss, Fisher, Deming, Bradford Hill and Cochrane.

April 1997
Richard Jones and Brian Payne

ACKNOWLEDGEMENTS

The authors are grateful to the following for permission to reproduce or adapt material for certain figures used in this publication.

Cambridge University Press. The Life, Letters and Labours of Francis Galton by Karl Pearson, 1930 (Cover Plate).

Elsevier/North Holland Biomedical Press, Philips S D *et al*, *Clin Chim Acta* 1978; **89**: 71-8 (Figure 1.13).

BMJ Publishing Group, Payne R B, *Br Med J* 1978; **1**: 22 (Figure 1.14), Chisholm A, *Br Med J* 1996; **312**: 931 (Figure 4.5).

Little, Brown and Company, Boston, Sackett D L *et al*, *Clinical Epidemiology: a Basic Science for Clinical Medicine* 2nd edn, 1991 (Figure 3.34).

The authors are grateful to Mrs Win Barney for her expert help with the manuscript and are particularly grateful to Sally Hollis of Lancaster University, Statistics Editor of the Annals of Clinical Biochemistry and to Dr Andrew Moore of Oxford University, Editor of Bandolier: Evidence-Based Health Care, for their helpful comments and corrections on a draft of this book. Any remaining errors and omissions are entirely the responsibility of the authors.

We should also like to acknowledge that the idea of a statistics book with few equations illustrating the application of computer programs arose during the course of many stimulating discussions about data interpretation with the late Professor Brian Morgan.

This book is dedicated to the memory of Stephen Walter

Contents

JOHANN KARL FRIEDRICH GAUSS

Born Brunswick 1777. Died Göttingen 1855.

Johann Gauss, the son of a gardener, was an infant prodigy in mathematics who was able to help his father with his accounts when he was only three years old. He made numerous discoveries in mathematics and astronomy, many of them while still a teenager. He studied mathematics at Göttingen University from 1795 - 1798, and for his doctoral thesis submitted a proof of the 'fundamental theorem of algebra' that had challenged mathematicians for centuries. His 1801 book, *Disquisitiones Arithmeticae*, remains a classical work. He was appointed Professor of Mathematics and Director of the Observatory in Göttingen in 1807, posts he retained until his death in 1855. At the Observatory he studied a variety of instruments and personally made many measurements. These studies led him to propose that observations were subject to a large number of small, independent errors and so would be "normally" distributed. Gauss had used Legendre's method of least squares as a student and was the first to connect it with the theory of probability. His work has been fundamental to the development of the whole of distribution-based statistics. In addition to his major work in mathematics and astronomy, Gauss made important discoveries in optics and in electricity and magnetism; the unit for magnetic field intensity is today called the gauss.

He was recognised as the greatest mathematician of his time even by Laplace, who was never free with compliments, and he was called the Prince of Mathematicians by his contemporaries. He has been judged by modern mathematicians to compare in stature with Archimedes and Newton; but in breadth to outstrip them both.

One criticism that might be levelled at him is that he did not publish his discoveries promptly. As a result, a number of mathematicians were chagrined to find that discoveries they made after his death (and for which they were honoured) had already been described by Gauss in unpublished papers.

Chapter 1

Statistical questions and kinds of data

WHY ARE STATISTICS USED?

Patients may respond very differently to exactly the same dose of a drug, and not everyone who smokes large numbers of cigarettes develops lung cancer. It is fairly unusual to find that a patient's pulse rate or blood pressure is exactly the same when the measurement is repeated, even if only a few minutes later, and a repeated laboratory investigation rarely gives exactly the same result. Even repeated analyses of the same sample will give a range of different results, albeit a narrow one. Biological and analytical variations like these can confuse the interpretation of data and obscure important underlying real effects.

The immense value of statistical methods is that they are able to dissect variability away and thus reveal any real effect which may underlie the noise. In addition to this primary role, many statistical methods are also able to provide quantitative data about the size and likely limits of an effect. Conversely, in situations where the variability of observations is predictable, statistical methods can help with the design of investigations by calculating the minimum number of observations needed to detect an underlying effect of specified size.

WHAT QUESTIONS ARE ASKED AND HOW ARE RESULTS EXPRESSED?

DIFFERENCE, CHANGE AND ASSOCIATION

Three main statistical questions are asked of data. The first is whether two or more groups of observations differ from each other. The second is whether observations have changed when repeated on a subsequent occasion. The third is whether there is an underlying association between different observations or measurements which may have been made at the same time.

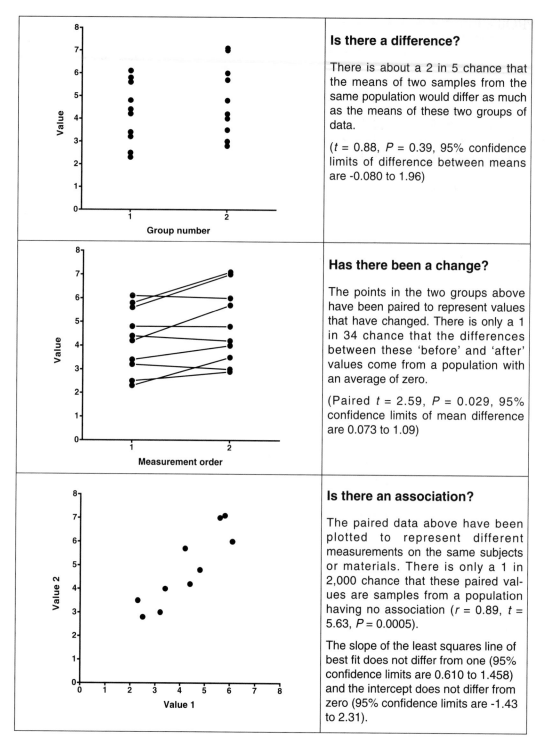

Is there a difference?

There is about a 2 in 5 chance that the means of two samples from the same population would differ as much as the means of these two groups of data.

($t = 0.88$, $P = 0.39$, 95% confidence limits of difference between means are -0.080 to 1.96)

Has there been a change?

The points in the two groups above have been paired to represent values that have changed. There is only a 1 in 34 chance that the differences between these 'before' and 'after' values come from a population with an average of zero.

(Paired $t = 2.59$, $P = 0.029$, 95% confidence limits of mean difference are 0.073 to 1.09)

Is there an association?

The paired data above have been plotted to represent different measurements on the same subjects or materials. There is only a 1 in 2,000 chance that these paired values are samples from a population having no association ($r = 0.89$, $t = 5.63$, $P = 0.0005$).

The slope of the least squares line of best fit does not differ from one (95% confidence limits are 0.610 to 1.458) and the intercept does not differ from zero (95% confidence limits are -1.43 to 2.31).

Figure 1.1 Difference, change and association

PROBABILITY

"But to us, probability is the very guide of life"
Bishop Butler (1692-1752)
The Analogy of Religion

All statistical tests calculate the probability that an observed difference, change or association has occurred by chance and can be accounted for by the variability in the observations. The tests examine the hypothesis that the observations are a sample from a population that shows no real difference, change or association. This hypothesis is called the 'null hypothesis' and is the opposite of the 'research hypothesis' that leads to the observations being made in the first place. The probability that the null hypothesis is true is given on a scale from 0 to 1. An answer of 0 implies that there really is a difference or association; an answer of 1 implies that there is no difference or association. So if the probability value is small we reject the null hypothesis and accept the research hypothesis. Probability (P) is sometimes expressed as a percentage, so that a value of 0.05 may be written as 5% and a value of 0.01 as 1%.

The smaller the probability value, the greater the 'statistical significance' is said to be. It should be remembered that statistical significance is not necessarily the same thing as practical or clinical significance; a "statistically significant" finding may be of little or no importance. For example, a statistically significant mean difference of 0.004 mmol/L that was found between measured ionized calcium values in the same blood samples taken into plain and into SST tubes was of no practical importance; normal values lie between 1.14 and 1.28 mmol/L and clinically important values deviate widely from this range.

If an experiment were designed to find out whether a new and an old brand of pipette differ in the repeatability with which they deliver plasma, the null hypothesis would be that they are equally reproducible. If statistical analysis of the data gave $P = 0.05$, the chance of finding the observed difference if the null hypothesis were true is only 5% or 1 in 20, a value often taken somewhat arbitrarily as the upper limit of statistical significance. Another way of looking at this result is that if one made measurements on an infinite number of new and old brand pipettes which really did not differ in reproducibility, there is a 1 in 20 chance that a sample of the same size would show the same difference.

ONE-TAILED AND TWO-TAILED TESTS
When differences between two sets of data are to be examined one should be clear before starting data collection whether the research hypothesis, the converse of the null hypothesis, is that the groups differ in *either* direction (needing what is called a two-tailed test) or that there is a difference in a *specified* direction (needing a one-tailed test). For the same data and the identical statistical calculation, the one-tailed probability is usually half the two-tailed probability. The concept of one- and two-sided tests does not apply when more than two groups are being compared.

The experiment with two brands of pipette described above is more likely to have been designed to find out whether the new brand is more reproducible than the old brand rather than whether there is any difference at all between brands. The null hypothesis therefore becomes that there is no difference *or* that the new pipettes are less reproducible than the old. If the two-tailed probability is 0.05 and the new brand *is* more reproducible than the old, the one-tailed probability is 0.025.

There has been controversy among statisticians about whether there is often real justification for using the directional one-sided test, largely because any significant difference may prove to be of interest whatever the null hypothesis. Most recommend that a two-sided test is used as a matter of course. If a one-tailed probability is reported, its use should be fully justified.

CONFIDENCE INTERVALS

> "...in confidence shall be your strength"
>
> *Isaiah* 30:15

A confidence interval gives a measure of the uncertainty inherent in a study in absolute units. A single set of measured data is an imprecise estimate of the larger population of which it is a sample, so all calculated values based on the sample have their own inherent imprecision. If the mean sodium concentration in serum from a sample of 100 blood donors were 140 mmol/L, calculation of its confidence interval might reveal that the true mean in all blood donors had a 95% probability ($P = 0.95$) of lying between 139.5 and 140.5 mmol/L. In other words, we can be confident that 95% of the means of samples of the same size from an infinitely large group of blood donors would lie within these limits. If the blood donor mean were compared with a mean in a group of patients of 138 mmol/L and a 95% confidence interval of 137.5 to 138.5 mmol/L, the absence of overlap of the ranges encompassing the true means would be apparent. Thus, it would be very unlikely the samples had come from the same population, even though the two sets of measured data themselves would overlap considerably.

Confidence intervals have the advantage over probability values of providing quantitative information about the variability of calculated values and the magnitude of differences or changes. The International Committee of Medical Journal Editors now expects authors of scientific papers to give confidence intervals in addition to, or instead of, probability (P) values whenever possible.

WHAT KINDS OF DATA CAN BE TESTED?

Which statistical tests can be applied to answer a question about a difference, a change or an association depends critically on the nature of the data that have been collected. Data are obtained in one of three ways:

- by classification into unrelated categories
- by ranking into series
- by measurement

CLASSIFIED DATA

Classified data (also called nominal data) are obtained by counting the numbers of observations falling into two or more unrelated categories. For example, in an absolute differential white count, white blood cells may be classified as neutrophils, lymphocytes, monocytes, eosinophils or basophils. Similarly, patients may be classified into groups according to their ethnic origin.

Among the tests that can be applied to classified data are the exact probability test of Fisher (page 6) for associations between classifications in a two by two table, the chi-squared (χ^2) test (page 61) for associations between rows and columns for larger independent classifications and McNemar's χ^2 test (page 60) to examine paired data for changes in classification.

As an example of classified data, in an investigation of symptoms in hospital patients it was found that anorexia was complained of by 38 of 64 patients with hypercalcaemia due to malignancy but only 18 of 48 with similar degrees of hypercalcaemia due to hyperparathyroidism.

	Malignancy	Hyperparathyroidism	Totals
Anorexia	38	18	56
No anorexia	26	30	56
Totals	64	48	112

Figure 1.2 Classification of anorexia by cause of hypercalcaemia

The null hypothesis is that the sample is from a population with the same proportion of patients with anorexia in each diagnostic category, in this case, 56 (38 + 18) out of 112 (64 + 48) or 50%. Fisher's exact probability test for a two by two table gave $P = 0.035$ or 3.5%. It was thus unlikely that the anorexia in the hypercalcaemic patients with malignancy could be entirely attributed to their hypercalcaemia.

FISHER'S EXACT PROBABILITY TEST

Application

Fisher's exact test is applied to a two by two frequency table of classified data to test the null hypothesis that there is no relation between the frequencies in the rows and the columns.

Requirements

The observations must be independent, that is, individual subjects must appear in only one of the four cells and must not be matched in any way with subjects in another cell. Patients before and after treatment, for example, or patients and closely matched individual controls are not independent and McNemar's χ^2 test for paired data should be used instead. In Fisher's test there is no lower limit to the number of observations in any of the four cells.

Basis of the calculation

The calculation of exact probability uses the products of factorials, so before the days of computers it could be very tedious for more than small numbers (Factorial 9 (9!) is, for example, $9 \times 8 \times 7 \times 6 \times 5 \times 4 \times 3 \times 2 = 362,880$). The only limitation nowadays is the capacity of the computer software and hardware that is used.

The product of the factorials of the marginal totals is divided by the product of the factorials of the total number and the frequencies in each of the cells to give the probability of the observed classification table. To this is added the calculated probabilities of all the more extreme tables with the same column and row totals. The latter are obtained by successively reducing the frequency in the smallest cell by one until zero is reached while keeping the marginal totals constant.

Interpretation

The test result is the exact probability that the observed frequencies or any more extreme frequencies would occur by chance if row and column frequencies were not related. (The probability of obtaining a distribution *less* extreme than the one observed if the null hypothesis were true is one minus the calculated probability. This is because one of all the possible classification tables must occur, so the probabilities of all possible combinations must add up to one.)

Figure 1.3 Fisher's exact probability test

RANKED DATA

Ranked data (also called ordinal data) are obtained by counting the numbers of observations falling into categories that form an ordered sequence. For example, the number of results of a urine dipstick test that are classified as negative, +, ++, +++ or ++++ form ranked data. The ranking is usually made on the basis of some kind of semiquantitive measurement or on an assessment score, such as the classification of the severity of post-operative pain as absent, mild, moderate or severe, but it can also be based on other kinds of series. If immature white cells were present in a blood specimen, counts of blast cells, promyelocytes, myelocytes and metamyelocytes would also comprise ranked data.

Among the statistical tests that can be applied to ranked data are the Mann-Whitney U-test, sometimes called the Wilcoxon-Mann-Whitney U-test, (page 8) for differences between two independent samples, Kruskal-Wallis' one-way analysis of variance for differences between more than two independent samples, Friedman's two-way analysis of variance for differences between matched groups studied under different conditions and the Wilcoxon matched-pairs signed-ranks test (page 62) for changes in ranking. In addition, association between pairs of variables can be tested by calculating the Spearman or Kendall rank correlation coefficient. These tests and their use are summarised in Figure 4.11 (page 146).

The null hypothesis of each of these tests is that the data are samples from the same infinitely large population of ranked data. If the observations are not themselves in numerical form, each ascending rank must be ascribed an ascending numerical value. For example, each result of a series of urine dipstick tests reported as negative, +, ++, +++ and ++++ might be assigned a value of 1, 2, 3, 4 or 5 or, indeed, any other ordered sequence of numbers such as 0, 6, 38, 150 or 999.

The tests are also applied to measured data when they do not fulfil the criteria that are discussed below which allow 'parametric' tests to be used (page 9). For example, if data were collected on the length of times taken to report emergency analyses before and after the introduction of new analytical equipment, it might well be found that neither group of data fulfils the parametric criteria and neither can be 'transformed' (page 16) to do so. The Mann-Whitney U-test would then be an appropriate test to find out whether analysis time had changed.

MANN-WHITNEY *U*-TEST

Application

The Mann-Whitney *U*-test is applied to two groups of independent ranked data to test the null hypothesis that they are samples from the same population of ranked data.

Requirements

The groups of ranked observations must be independent. If this is not the case, for example, ranked symptoms in the same patients before and after treatment or ranked observations in patients and individually closely matched controls, then Wilcoxon's matched-pairs signed-ranks test should be used instead.

Mechanics of the calculation

The observations in both groups are ranked together, assigning increasing numerical values to the ranks, and assigning tied observations the average of the values of the tied ranks. The statistic *U* is the number of times that a ranking in the group with the larger number of observations (if there is one) precedes a ranking in the other group.

Interpretation

Most computer programs give the probability derived from the value of *U* of obtaining the observed difference if the two groups are samples from the same population. If the probability is not given, it can be read from tables for small numbers or calculated when there are more than twenty observations in the larger group (see Siegel and Castellan (1988), *Nonparametric Statistics for the Behavioral Sciences*).

Figure 1.4 Mann-Whitney *U*-test

MEASURED DATA

Measured data (also called interval or continuous data) form the bulk of the observations in clinical and laboratory medicine that require statistical analysis. They are recorded in conventional units such as mmol/L, kPa or cells/mm.

PARAMETRIC TESTS

The tests that can be applied to measured data include all the tests listed above under ranked data together with some rather more powerful tests, called parametric tests, that should be applied only if the measured data fulfil certain criteria that are described below. 'Parameters' are quantities such as the standard deviation that are used to define theoretical distributions, so distribution-based statistical tests are called parametric tests. Both parametric and non-parametric (distribution-free) statistical tests are able to provide probability values for a difference, a change or an association and also confidence intervals for positional values like the mean of measured data or the median of ranked data (the value with an equal number of observations above and below it). Parametric tests have the advantages that only they are able to define mathematically the relationship between associated variables and provide confidence intervals for that relationship.

Among parametric tests are the *F*-test for differences in·scatter (page 31) and the *t*-test for differences in means between two samples (page 40), one-way analysis of variance to test for differences between more than two samples (page 33), two-way analysis of variance for differences between matched groups studied under different conditions, the paired *t*-test to assess change (page 59) and Pearson correlation and least-squares linear regression to describe association (page 52).

WHEN CAN PARAMETRIC TESTS BE USED?

THE NORMAL DISTRIBUTION

The fundamental assumption of parametric tests such as the *F*-test and the *t*-test is that the data are a sample from a large population which has a Gaussian or 'Normal' distribution. Karl Friedrich Gauss proposed the distribution to describe the random component of repeated measurements of the same thing. The concept was subsequently extended by the Belgian astronomer Adolphe Quetelet to describe the variation of ·measurements of biological variables *between* subjects.

Some think that the title 'the Gaussian curve' gives undue credit to one man and that it would be better called 'the curve of De Moivre, Bernouilli, Laplace and Gauss.' It is a characteristic of scientific discovery that it may be made simultaneously by independent workers; the Gaussian curve was described completely independently by A M Legendre in 1806. Because the potential title is inordinately long if credit is given to everyone, we have chosen to use the expression the 'Normal' curve in this book. Normal used in this way means 'standard' from the Latin *norma*, a carpenter's square.

STANDARD DEVIATION AND VARIANCE

The standard deviation (SD) of a Normal distribution is a measure of the scatter of observations about the mean in the same units as the observations themselves. It is the square root of the variance, which can be expressed in words as the mean of the squares of the differences between each value and the arithmetic mean of the measurements. (In practice the sum of squares is divided by one less than the number of observations to avoid a minor underestimation of the SD of the population of which the observations are a sample.)

Figure 1.5   Standard deviation and variance

If the measured values are plotted on the x axis and the number of observations at each value on the y axis, a Normal distribution is symmetrical and bell-shaped with the mean at the highest point (the mode).

In a true Normal distribution the proportion of values falling within multiples of SDs from the mean can be predicted. For example:

- 68.2% of values fall within plus and minus one SD
- 95.5% of values fall within plus and minus two SDs
- 99.7% of values fall within plus and minus three SDs

(Exactly 95% of values fall within the mean plus and minus 1.96 SDs, with 2.5% of values above and 2.5% of values below this confidence interval.) However, while the Normal distribution is a very close approximation to the distribution both of measurement errors and of many biological variables between individuals, it cannot be exact because the theoretical bell-shaped curve never actually reaches the x axis but stretches to infinity in both directions.

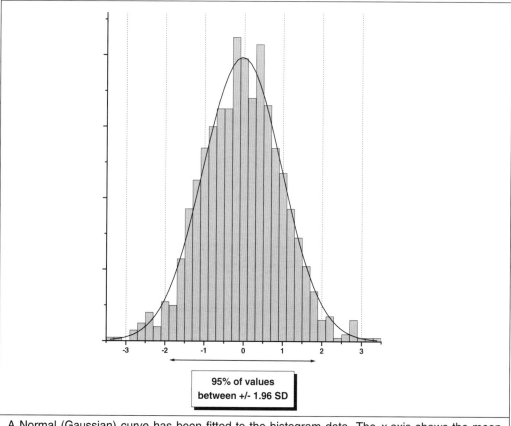

A Normal (Gaussian) curve has been fitted to the histogram data. The x axis shows the mean (0) and standard deviations from the mean.

Figure 1.6 The Normal distribution

HOW ARE THE DISTRIBUTIONS OF GROUP DATA ASSESSED?

Before a parametric test is applied to assess whether groups of data differ from each other, each group should first be inspected for divergence from a symmetrical bell-shaped Normal distribution and for data points which do not appear to belong to the bulk of the data - so-called outliers. To assess *changes* in a measurement the appropriate distribution to examine for Normality and outliers is that of the *differences* between the paired values; the distributions of the 'before' and 'after' samples are irrelevant in this case. The assumptions of the parametric test for association, least-squares linear regression, also involve the Normal distribution and are discussed below.

Parametric statistical analysis takes data to be a random sample from a much larger population of values with a smooth Normal distribution. However, visual interpretation of the ups and downs of a simple histogram of a small data set may be difficult, especially as histograms of the same data set can vary greatly in appearance when different measurement intervals are chosen for the x axis.

NORMAL PROBABILITY PLOT

A satisfactory visual way to judge Normality is provided by a Normal probability or probit plot. An appropriate computer program transforms measured values into standard Normal deviate values, sometimes known as Normal scores, by subtracting the mean and dividing by the standard deviation, and then ranks them in ascending order. A plot of the cumulative ranked scores from a true Normal distribution with a mean of zero and a standard deviation of one against the measured values gives a perfect straight line. If a computer program is not available, the cumulative frequency of observations at ascending measured values as a percentage of the total must be calculated and plotted against the values themselves on Normal probability graph paper.

The eye is good at recognising straight lines, and usually visual inspection for linearity of the plot is all that is necessary. A useful tip is to pick up the paper on which the plot is drawn and tilt it so that one is looking along the line. When this is done slight non-linearity becomes much more obvious. Minor deviations from linearity at the upper and lower ends of the line are usually of no consequence if the centre portion is clearly linear.

Figure 1.7   Normal probability plot

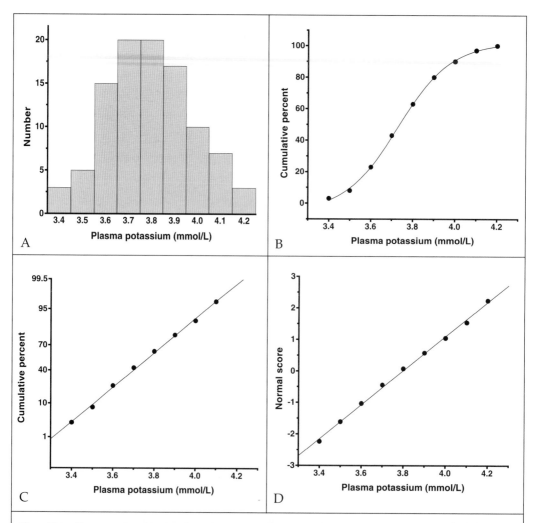

The 100 plasma potassium values in A have been plotted as cumulative percentages in B showing that, for example, 80% of values are 3.9 mmol/L or less and 90% are 4.0 mmol/L or less. The cumulative percent scale in C has been changed to a Normal probability scale to convert the sigmoid curve of a Normal distribution into a straight line. Probability graph paper with this scale can be used to plot data if a computer program is not available. In D the Normal probability scale has been converted to standard Normal deviates or Normal scores.

Figure 1.8   Normal probability plotting to test Normality

MATHEMATICAL TESTS FOR NORMALITY

Confirmation that a distribution differs significantly from a Normal one can be obtained mathematically. There is little point in carrying out such calculations if numbers are small, say less than 30, and the Normal probability plot gives a reasonably straight line. No mathematical test is perfect in this regard, but a number are commonly used or are recommended by official bodies such as the International Federation of Clinical Chemistry (IFCC). However, with large sample sizes, very small deviations from Normality will be statistically significant.

Skewness indicates the degree of asymmetry of a distribution. For a Normal distribution the value is zero. Left tail (negative) skew gives a value less than zero and right tail (positive) skew a value greater than zero.

Kurtosis is a measure of the 'peakiness' of a distribution, departure from Normality occurring with either tall-thin or low-flat samples. For a Normal distribution a value of 3 is expected. Values greater than 3 indicate peakiness and values less than 3 squatness. Formal tests of Normality include the Anderson Darling test and the Kolmogorov-Smirnov test. Both are non-parametric distribution function tests that examine the fit of the observed distribution to a Normal distribution. Other tests include the Shapiro Wilks *W* test and the Shapiro Francia *W'* test which are discussed by Altman (1991) in *Practical Statistics for Medical Research* (see Further Reading).

All four tests produce a probability value, and there is a question about what order of magnitude of probability is important in deciding whether one is able to use the data for parametric statistical tests. Parametric tests are said to be 'robust' because minor deviations from Normality have little effect on their results. As a rule of thumb, it is reasonable to use parametric methods if the tests for Normality give probability values of 0.1 or greater.

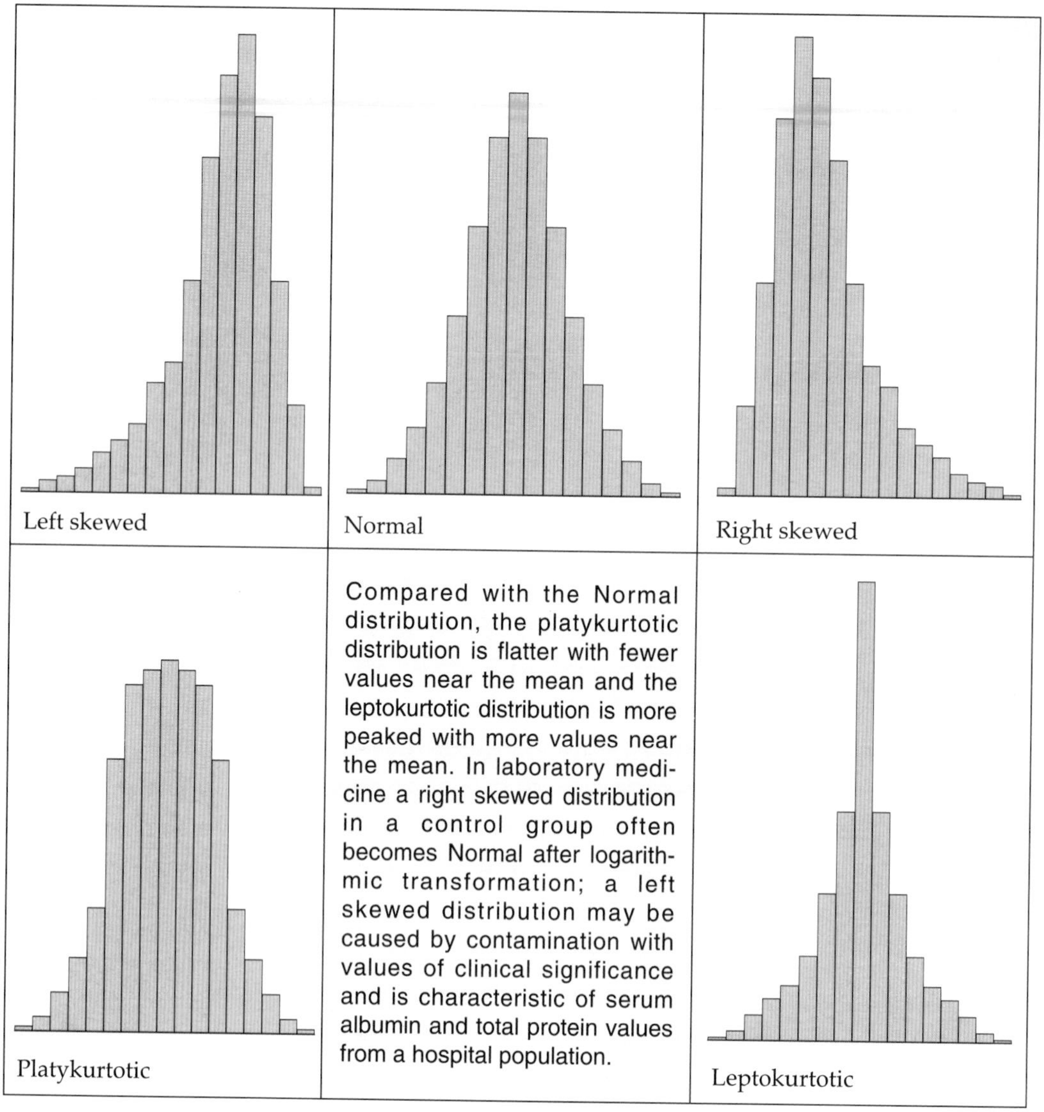
Left skewed
Normal
Right skewed
Platykurtotic
Compared with the Normal distribution, the platykurtotic distribution is flatter with fewer values near the mean and the leptokurtotic distribution is more peaked with more values near the mean. In laboratory medicine a right skewed distribution in a control group often becomes Normal after logarithmic transformation; a left skewed distribution may be caused by contamination with values of clinical significance and is characteristic of serum albumin and total protein values from a hospital population.
Leptokurtotic

Figure 1.9 Normal, kurtotic and right and left skewed distributions

WHAT CAN BE DONE WITH NON-NORMAL GROUPED DATA OR DIFFERENCES?

The most common reason for measured clinical data to produce a curved line on a Normal probability plot which is concave towards the concentration axis and to fail the tests for Normality is that they have a log-Normal distribution, skewed to the right with a tail of high values. If logarithms of the measured values are plotted and used in the calculations, the criteria for Normality are fulfilled. This 'transformation' of the data to logarithms allows parametric tests to be carried out and quantitative data, including confidence intervals, to be obtained.

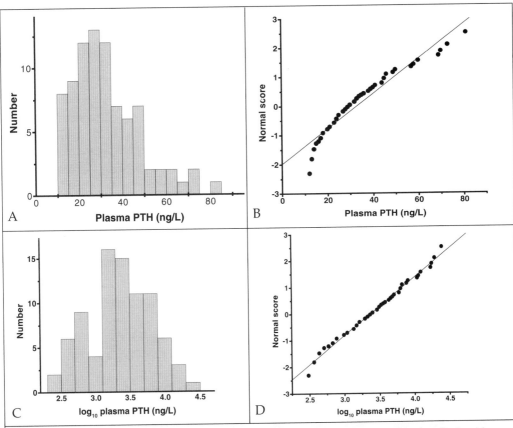

The histogram of 84 plasma PTH values from patients with no clinical or biochemical evidence of a disturbance of calcium homeostasis in A appears skewed to the right and the cumulative percent values plotted as Normal scores in B are curved towards the concentration axis. The histogram of the logarithms of the values in C is symmetrical and the Normal scores fall on a straight line D. The logarithms show a Normal distribution so, if a computer program were not available, the 95.5% confidence limits of the sample could be determined by taking the antilogarithms of the values where Normal scores of +2 and -2 intersect the line.

Figure 1.10 Logarithmic transformation

TRANSFORMATIONS

Logarithmic transformation is by far the most important form of transformation for data in clinical and laboratory medicine. When measured values approach zero (for example, the activity of many serum enzymes in health) a log distribution is almost inevitably produced, while observations clustered around a physiologically controlled point away from zero (for example, serum sodium or potassium concentrations) can equally well be described by a Normal or a log-Normal distribution. Some have advocated that biological data should be log-transformed as a matter of course. Peter Oldham in his book *Measurement in Medicine* (1968) pointed out that if the distribution of the size of cherries were determined by factors that act in a multiplicative way like the logarithmic scale, then the logarithms of their volumes, surface areas and diameters would all be Normally distributed. Transformation to any base is equally effective, for example, common logarithms to the base 10 ($\log_{10}$) or natural logarithms to the base e ($\log_e$). Titres are log-distributed and can be transformed simply by replacing the dilutions such as 1 in 2, 4, 8, 16 and so on by the numbers 1, 2, 3, 4 and so on, effectively transforming them to logarithms to the base 2 ($\log_2$).

Other transformations, such as reciprocal, square root, square and cube can also be used but are only rarely of value in clinical practice. Logarithmically transformed data can be back-transformed after statistical calculations to provide, for example, confidence intervals in the original units of measurement. A disadvantage of other transformations is that back-transformation cannot produce meaningful results.

Parametric tests involving means can be applied without further investigation of the distribution and without transformation if a sufficiently large number of data points is available, because with large numbers the means are Normally distributed whatever the distribution of data points (the 'Central Limit Theorem'). However, it is not possible to calculate, for example, parametric confidence limits from the sample in such a situation, so transformation is generally preferable.

If transformation of measured data fails to change them to a Normal distribution, and numbers are not large, non-parametric tests such as the Mann-Whitney U-test for differences between two independent samples or the Wilcoxon matched-pairs signed-ranks test for changes must be used. However, it is still possible to calculate confidence intervals for the median of a data set and for such other 'positional' quantities as, for example, the 5th and 95th centiles (see Gardner and Altman (1989), *Statistics with Confidence: Confidence Intervals and Statistical Guidelines*).

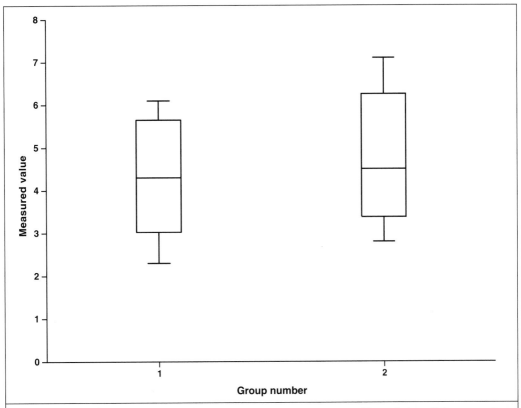

A box and whisker plot is a convenient way of representing non-Normal data if there are too many points to display as a scattergram. The central line is the median (the value with an equal number of observations above and below it). The box represents the central 50% of the data, limited by the 25th and 75th percentiles. The limits of the whiskers may show either the extreme values or the 2.5% and 97.5% values.

Figure 1.11 Box and whisker plot to describe non-Normal data

HOW IS THE NORMALITY OF REGRESSION DATA ASSESSED?

The assumptions of the parametric test for association, least-squares linear regression, are that there is a straight line which can be drawn through the means of the x and y values in such a way that the data points have a Normal distribution about it in the y direction at each value of x, and that the SDs of y are similar at all values of x. The simplest way to make a qualitative assessment of whether the data are distributed in this way is to plot them.

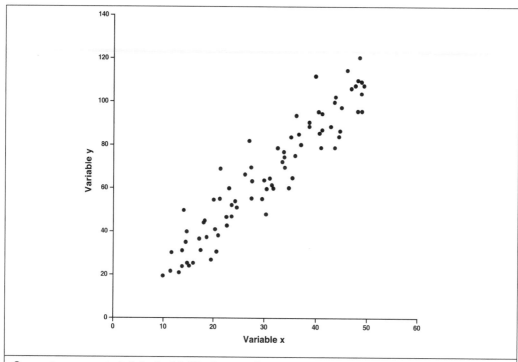

Computer-generated data that fulfils the requirements for least squares linear regression: a linear relationship between the variables with a Normal distribution of *y* values at each value of *x*.

Figure 1.12   Ideal linear regression data

If no clear pattern emerges there is usually little practical point in going further. Sometimes a relationship can be seen, but the scatter is so wide that no useful prediction could be made of *y* from *x* as is the case, for example, if one examines the relationship between plasma urea and plasma creatinine concentrations in hospital patients. At the opposite extreme, when all the points lie very close to a straight line - for example, when the optical densities developed in a chemical analytical method are plotted against the concentration of the substance being measured - there is no need to assess Normality.

WHAT CAN BE DONE WITH NON-NORMAL REGRESSION DATA?

If the cloud of data points appears to show a relationship, but one of the variables has more low and fewer high values at each value of the other, logarithmic transformation of that variable may be helpful. For example, when urine oestriol excretion was plotted against week of normal pregnancy from weeks thirty-two to thirty-eight, oestriol excretion values were clearly skewed with more low and fewer high values. Transformation to logarithms resulted in a more symmetrical distribution about a straight line and parametric least squares regression could then be used.

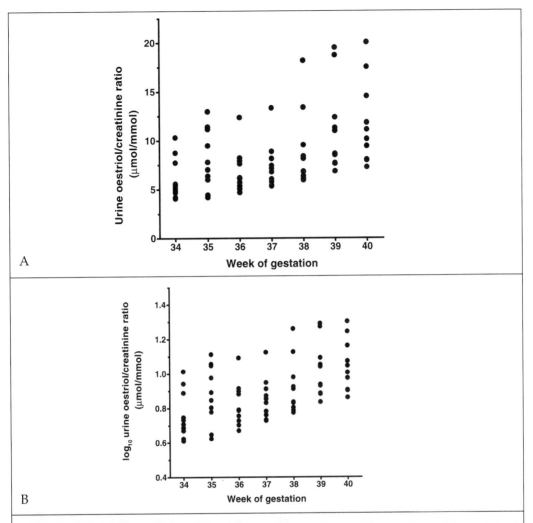

The urine oestriol/creatinine ratio in first morning urine specimens increases through normal pregnancy but shows a logarithmic distribution at each week (A). Transformation of the ratios to logarithms (B) allows the application of least squares regression.

From: Philips S D, Salway J G, Payne R B, MacDonald H N. Interpretation of urinary oestrogen-creatinine ratio for monitoring feto-placental function in late pregnancy. *Clin Chim Acta* 1978; **89**: 71-8

Figures 1.13 Semi-log regression data

Similarly, it sometimes looks as though the best line through the cloud of points is curved and the spread of values of both variables increase together. An example of this is the relationship between the clearance of amylase and the clearance of creatinine in patients with varying degrees of renal failure. (Ratios of measured values are often logarithmically distributed.) When the logarithms of *both* variables were plotted, the distribution again became symmetrical about a straight line. The implication of such a finding is that the relationship between the variables is proportional so that, for example, a doubling of one variable might be associated with a three-fold increase in the other.

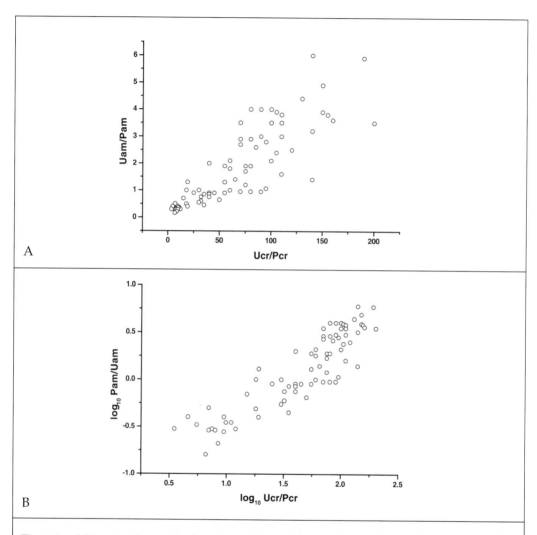

A

B

The ratio of the urine clearance of amylase to that of creatinine has been used for the retrospective diagnosis of acute pancreatitis. Reference data from normal subjects and patients with varying degrees of renal failure, A shows diverging points. Logarithmic transformation of both axes B gives 'ideal' regression data that allows the calculation of a reference interval for the ratio. U_{cr} = Urine creatinine, P_{cr} = Plasma creatinine, U_{am} = Urine amylase, P_{am} = Plasma amylase

From: Payne R B. Interpretation of amylase clearance in patients with abnormal creatinine clearance. *Br Med J* 1978; **i:** 22

Figures 1.14   Log:log regression data

Occasionally things can be improved a little by other transformations. For example, taking logarithms after the addition or subtraction of a constant might be applied if there appeared to be a curved relationship with an intercept on one of the axes. In this case it would be reasonable to subtract an approximate intercept value before transforming both sets of data to logarithms. (The optimum value could be found using an iterative computer program, but an approximation is better than nothing.) Oldham gives examples of other transformations: squaring the measured diameters of tuberculin reactions linearised their relationship with log dose of tuberculin because it effectively converted them to areas; and taking the reciprocal of airways resistance measurements (and so converting them to conductances) linearised their relationship with lung volume.

If no transformation produces a symmetrical scatter about a straight line, then the non-parametric Spearman or Kendall rank correlation coefficient can be calculated to assess the null hypothesis that there is no association. However, such data cannot be used to describe the nature of an association quantitatively, to predict the value of one variable from that of the other nor, of course, to calculate the confidence interval of the prediction.

WHEN SHOULD NON-PARAMETRIC TESTS BE USED FOR MEASURED DATA?

Non-parametric tests make no assumptions about the distribution of the population of which the observations are a sample, and so are used when the data are not Normally distributed and cannot be transformed to be so. An exception is that the parametric t-test for differences between means can be applied whatever the shape of the distributions if the numbers of observations are sufficiently large (page 40).

The t-test should not be used to compare the means of two small groups of data even though they are both Normally distributed if their variances differ significantly by the F-Test (page 31); the non-parametric Mann-Whitney U-test (page 8) should be used instead.

Finally, non-parametric methods must be used if some data points fall outside the limits of accurate measurement. Examples are data sets with a number of values for plasma glucose reported as 'less than 0.3 mmol/L' or with some values for plasma creatine kinase reported as 'greater than 10,000 IU/L'.

HOW IS DATA INPUT CHECKED?

It is critical that results are accurately transferred from the data sheets or work books in which they were collected into the computer. Data input should always be checked before values are plotted and calculations carried out. Transcription errors are common and easy to make, and a little effort here can avoid puzzling problems later in the analysis. When numbers are relatively small, say less than 200, checking is conveniently done by calling from the computer screen to a colleague reading the primary data. This becomes tedious and therefore prone to errors with large numbers of results, so there is then really no alternative to double entry of the data and checking that all the differences between the two data sets are zero. In some circumstances data may have been automatically transferred from another computer database. The values still need to be checked carefully because frame shifts or misreads can seriously disrupt data sets.

In addition to calling and reading or double entry, checks for classified data can include looking for impossible categories. For example, if males are entered as 1 and females as 2, no values above 2 are possible. Similarly for measured data, checks can be made for highly improbable values such as serum sodium concentrations less than 100 mmol/L or greater than 160 mmol/L. Range checks of this kind are useful in picking up omitted or shifted decimal points which are occasionally misread from the screen. Range checks can be applied to calculated results which will be analysed statistically as well as to primary data. For example, in addition to checking the plasma and urine concentrations of a substance and the timed urine volumes, the calculated renal clearances could also be subjected to a range check.

HOW ARE OUTLIERS DEALT WITH?

Having ensured as far as possible that transcription errors have been avoided, grouped data or differences should be examined as histograms and as Normal probability plots, and data that is to be tested for association should be examined as x-y plots. Outliers are defined as ranked or measured values that appear not to belong to the bulk of the data set. They are of particular importance for calculations with measured data because they have a large influence on both the mean value and the SD of Normal distributions and on regression coefficients.

If the histogram is skewed to the right with a small proportion of high outliers and the probability plot shows a curve that is concave towards the concentration axis, it is likely that a logarithmic transformation is needed and the apparent outliers are part of a logarithmic distribution. The possible transformation of either one or both variables that are to be examined for association has been discussed above (page 16).

Are there any hard criteria which allow outliers to be recognised? William Chauvenet, author of the *Manual of Spherical and Practical Astronomy* (1863), suggested that for measurements with an underlying Normal distribution, depending on the number of observations, values lying above or below a specified number of SDs from the mean might reasonably be considered to be unlikely to belong to the bulk of the data. Chauvenet's criterion is based on a linear relationship between the logarithm of the number of observations and their variance (SD^2). Some values are given in Figure 1.15.

Number of observations	Limiting number of standard deviations from the mean
10	1.96
20	2.24
30	2.39
40	2.50
50	2.58
100	2.80
200	3.02
500	3.29

Figure 1.15 Some values that meet Chauvenet's criterion

It is our view that Chauvenet's criterion, or any other mathematical criterion, should not be used to exclude values but rather to direct attention to values that need further examination. The possibilities that then need to be considered in clinical and laboratory medicine include:

- *Blunders.* Gross errors, such as analysing the wrong sample or using a wrong size pipette, can usually be checked by repeating the measurement. Automation of laboratory procedures together with computerisation has reduced but by no means eliminated blunders. It should be noted that repeating a measurement on a specimen taken from the wrong patient or labelled with the wrong patient's identification in the laboratory will not detect the blunder. A fresh specimen from the patient is needed.

- *Inadequate sample mixing.* The dangers of making haematological measurements without adequate mixing of the sample, particularly if the sedimentation rate is high, are self-evident. Less obvious is the layering that is present in an unmixed thawed serum or plasma sample; proteins and substances bound to them are present in much higher concentration at the bottom of the sample than at the top.

- *Short sampling.* Sophisticated automated analytical equipment can often warn of inadequate specimen volume, but even in the presence of such a system spuriously low values can be produced. If that proves to be the case for the outlier by repeat analysis, all residual samples should also be examined for possible short sampling.

- *Partially blocked sample probe.* Fibrinogen particles may appear in antico-agulated samples particularly if they are frozen and thawed before analysis and cause short sampling.

- *Analytical interference.* Some methods on some analytical instruments are susceptible to interference, usually giving spuriously high values in the presence of jaundice, haemolysis or hyperlipidaemia in the sample. If that is the case, not only the outlier but all the samples should be examined.

- *Transcription errors.* Ways of minimising these during computer input have been discussed above but transcriptions are also made from, for example, the displays of measuring equipment. About 0.5% of transcriptions are said to be likely to be incorrect, so the fewer steps between a measurement being made and the data being recorded in the computer the better. In clinical pathology, direct links between measuring instruments and the laboratory computer have reduced the transcription error rate considerably.

- *Unsuspected disease.* When data are being collected from apparently healthy individuals to construct a reference range for use in diagnosis, an outlying value may represent the effect of a disease process before it has become clinically manifest. Because further investigation of the subject to confirm this hypothesis may pose major ethical problems, it is wise to exclude all the above possibilities before proceeding.

If there are compelling logical or common-sense reasons, for example a value 7 SDs above the mean, then outliers should, of course, be eliminated. If no reason can be found, then that should be reported and the data analysed with and without the inclusion of outliers. This is particularly important when data are being examined for association. A single outlying pair of points can transform a cluster showing no relationship into an apparently 'significant' regression.

SUMMARY

Statistical tests are used to assess whether an apparent difference, change or association in classified, ranked or measured data is likely to be real or to be due to biological and analytical 'noise'. Results are usually expressed as the one- or two-tailed probability of obtaining the data if the null hypothesis were true. Results should be given as confidence intervals as well as or instead of probability values whenever possible. The extent to which a 'statistically significant' result is of biological or clinical significance can then be judged.

Statistical tests based on the Normal distribution should be used when the assumption of that distribution is justified or when the data can be transformed to a Normal distribution. **It is difficult to overemphasise the critical importance of examining measured data groups graphically as Normal probability plots or scatter plots to identify outliers and to confirm distributions before undertaking statistical analysis.**

FURTHER READING

Altman D G. *Practical Statistics for Medical Research.* London: Chapman and Hall, 1991

Gardner M J, Altman D G. *Statistics with Confidence: Confidence Intervals and Statistical Guidelines.* London: British Medical Association, 1989

Kirkwood B R. *Essentials of Medical Statistics.* Oxford: Blackwell Scientific, 1988

Oldham P D. *Measurement in Medicine: the Interpretation of Numerical Data.* London: English Universities Press, 1968

Siegel S, Castellan N J, Jr. *Nonparametric Statistics for the Behavioral Sciences.* New York: McGraw-Hill, 1988

RONALD AYLMER FISHER

Born East Finchley 17 February 1890. Died Adelaide 29 July 1962.

As a schoolboy Fisher had the ability to solve mathematical problems entirely in his head. From Harrow he won a scholarship to Cambridge where he became interested in the mathematics of evolution and genetics. After graduating in 1913 he was awarded a year's studentship to study statistical mechanics, quantum theory and the theory of errors.

He was unable to serve in the Army during 1914-18 because of poor eyesight, instead teaching mathematics and physics at several schools. His paper proving that Darwin's theory of gradual evolution was entirely consistent with Mendelian inheritance was completed in 1914, but was rejected by referees and was not published until 1918. It introduced analysis of variance for the first time.

In 1919 he became statistician at the Rothamsted Experimental Station for agricultural research. At that time the need to make best estimates from available data, central to the work of Gauss, had been lost sight of, and the work of Gossett ('Student') about the errors of small samples had received little interest. Fisher remedied both these deficiencies and extended the work to more complex problems. His 1925 book *'Statistical Methods for Research Workers'* was the first to introduce the concept of randomisation in experimental design. He was elected FRS in 1929.

In 1933 he succeeded Karl Pearson as Galton Professor at University College, London and while there published *'The Design of Experiments'* and, with Frank Yates, *'Statistical Tables for Biological, Agricultural and Medical Research'*. In 1943 he was appointed to the Arthur Balfour Chair of Genetics in Cambridge. While there he solved the problem of the mode of inheritance of Rhesus blood groups. He retired in 1957 and then took a research fellowship in the Commonwealth Scientific and Industrial Research Organisation in Adelaide where he remained (between visits to many other parts of the world) until his death in 1962.

Fisher was a charming and stimulating man who was good company. He enjoyed scientific controversy but had a somewhat contentious spirit and a quick temper. He had an early interest in the eugenic improvement of the intelligence of the population, and was concerned that the birth rate was lower in those of higher intelligence. The Fishers made their own contribution: he and Eileen had eight children.

Chapter 2

Analytical methods: control and comparison

WHY IS STATISTICAL CONTROL NECESSARY?

> 'The state of statistical control is therefore the goal of all experimentation.'
> W E Deming
> in *Statistical Method from the Viewpoint of Quality Control*

Edwards Deming, in his introduction to W A Shewhart's book on statistical aspects of quality control, emphasised that one cannot make predictions by the statistical analysis of data if the data themselves are unstable. Parametric statistics assume that the data analysed are a representative sample of a universal population, and this population includes future data. Thus, there is little point in trying to establish a reference range, an action limit or a therapeutic window for a laboratory investigation, or in attempting to determine minimum significant changes in patients' results, when measurements drift over time or show varying reproducibility. Similarly, research results can be a guide to future action only if the methods of measurement employed are robust.

HOW IS THE PERFORMANCE OF AN ANALYTICAL METHOD DESCRIBED?

The most important aspects of methodological performance are:

- Imprecision
- Bias
- Analytical specificity
- Detection limit
- Analytical range

Imprecision is a measure of the closeness of a series of measurements of the same material.

Bias (or inaccuracy) is the difference between the mean of a series of measurements of the same material and the true value.

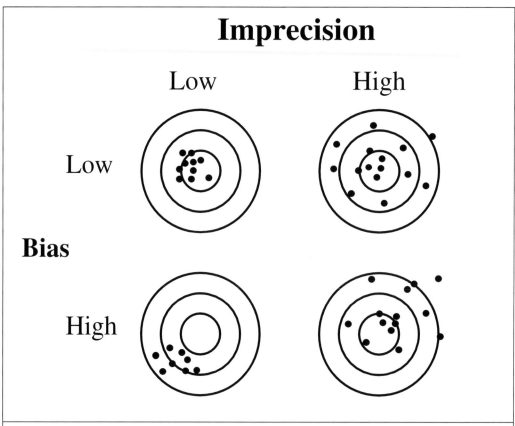

Imprecision

The bullseye represents the true target value and the points represent repeated measurements. The lower imprecision and bias, the closer a single measurement is likely to be to the target.

Figure 2.1 Imprecision and bias

Analytical specificity describes the extent to which other substances which may be present in a sample interfere with the analysis. It is usually expressed as the effect on the apparent measured concentration of given concentrations of the interfering endogenous or exogenous substance.

Detection limit is the smallest value that can be distinguished from zero with a defined degree of confidence.

The analytical range is simply the range of values that can be measured reproducibly. The lower limit may often be defined by the detection limit and the upper limit by an unacceptable increase in imprecision.

The definition of the 'method' includes such factors as the apparatus or instruments used as well as the reagents and the practical technique. Most journals that publish original work based on the statistical analysis of clinical measurements expect a literature reference to the method, details of modifications to reagents or operating procedures and information about the observed imprecision of the method at levels that are relevant to the investigation. The assessment of imprecision, bias and detection limit are considered in more detail below.

HOW IS IMPRECISION ASSESSED?

STANDARD DEVIATION AND COEFFICIENT OF VARIATION

Measurement error usually follows a Normal distribution. Imprecision is expressed as the standard deviation (SD) of repeated measurements of the same material. Alternatively, it may be expressed as the coefficient of variation (CV), which is simply the SD as a percentage of the mean value. CV is independent of the unit of measurement so that, for example, the CV would be the same whether partial pressure measurements were made in mmHg or kPa. Both SD and CV commonly differ with the size of the measured value, SD often increasing with concentration and CV falling. Some assays, particularly of hormones, show higher SDs at lower as well as at higher values with a U-shaped 'precision profile'. It is usual to determine the imprecision of clinical laboratory methods at values which are 'high', 'medium' and' low' in terms of clinically encountered results. In published work, the value or values at which imprecision was determined should always be stated.

The material measured to assess imprecision should resemble clinical material as closely as possible. Aqueous solutions, for example, often give SDs for common biochemical tests that are smaller than those given by serum. This possibility could be investigated formally for a new test by making repeated measurements of an aqueous solution and a serum with similar concentrations of analyte and testing whether the observed variances (SD^2) differed using the *F*-test, a test named in honour of R A Fisher.

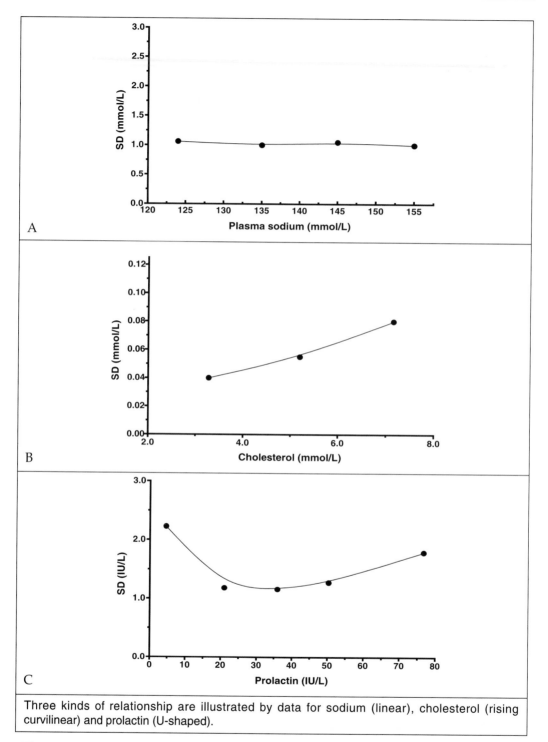

Three kinds of relationship are illustrated by data for sodium (linear), cholesterol (rising curvilinear) and prolactin (U-shaped).

Figure 2.2 Relationships between imprecision and value

THE *F*-TEST

Application

The *F*-test is applied to two groups of independent measurements to test the null hypothesis that their variances do not differ. It can be used to determine which kind of *t*-test could be applied to them. The *F*-test is an integral part of analysis of variance.

Requirements

Both groups of observations should have reasonably Normal distributions. This can be tested by inspecting Normal probability plots.

Basis of the calculation

The value *F* is simply the ratio of the larger to the smaller variance.

Interpretation

The probability that the variances would be observed in samples from the same population is derived from *F*. If the probability is not given by the computer program, a table of the distribution of *F* can be entered with its value and degrees of freedom one less than the number of observations in each of the samples taking care to enter degrees of freedom in the appropriate row or column.

Figure 2.3 The *F*-test

In spite of the fact that aqueous solutions generally have smaller imprecisions than plasma or serum specimens with similar concentrations, the imprecision of urine analyses may be greater than that of analyses of plasma or serum. This is because the concentrations of common analytes in urine are higher than in serum. As a consequence dilution is often necessary before analysis, introducing a pre-analytical source of variability, the diluting process. The basis of the Gaussian theory of the Normal distribution is that measurements are subject to a number of errors that are additive. In fact, it is the variances (SD^2) that have the important property of being additive, so that for example,

$$SD^2 = SD_a^2 + SD_b^2$$

Thus, when samples require dilution,

Measurement variance = true analytical variance + dilution variance

These equations can be remembered as the statistical equivalent of the theory of Pythagorus in geometry – in a right-angled triangle, the square of the hypotenuse (the combined variance) equals the sum of the squares on the other two sides (the variances of the contributing factors).

Clinical laboratory measurements are generally recorded to the number of significant figures that have proved to be useful in relation to the width of a reference range or to the magnitude of a clinically significant change. When assessing imprecision in a formal evaluation or method comparison, it is preferable to include a further significant figure whenever possible. There are two reasons for this. The first is that inspection of a histogram or a Normal probability plot to confirm that the data fulfil the requirements for parametric statistical analysis makes little sense when replicate analysis of, for example, a serum for its sodium or potassium concentration may give a spread of only three different values. The second is that the calculated SD or CV is always slightly larger the fewer the number of significant figures.

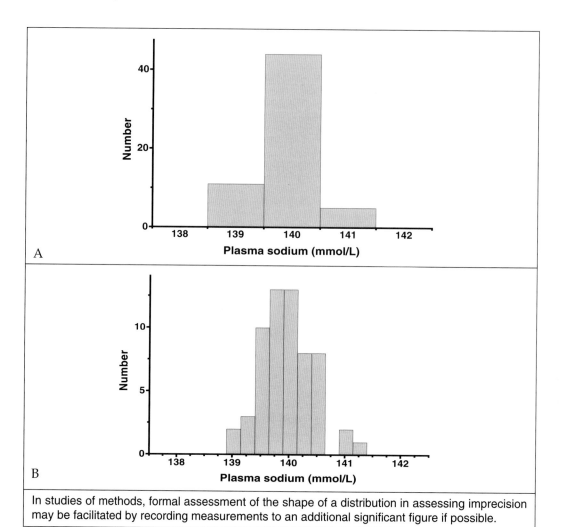

In studies of methods, formal assessment of the shape of a distribution in assessing imprecision may be facilitated by recording measurements to an additional significant figure if possible.

Figure 2.4 Effect of measurement interval on assessment of a distribution

Repeated measurement of the same material introduces the problem of time-related changes. In the early days of AutoAnalysers it was shown that the mean value of replicates analysed in different batches (analyser plates) on the same day or between days could change following recalibration. The question of whether one or more of a series of batches differs from the series as a whole could be investigated formally using one-way analysis of variance, making repeated measurements of the same material interspersed with recalibrations.

ONE-WAY ANALYSIS OF VARIANCE

Application

One-way analysis of variance is applied when differences are suspected between the means of a number of groups of observations to test the null hypothesis that the groups are samples from the same population.

Requirements

The groups should have reasonably Normal distributions with reasonably similar variances. The distributions can be inspected as Normal probability plots and the F_{max} test can be used to compare variances. In this test the largest variance is divided by the smallest; the significance of the ratio is found by entering a table of the cumulative probability of F_{max} with degrees of freedom one less than the number of observations in the smaller of the two groups and with the total number of groups. If the data do not fulfil these requirements and cannot be transformed to do so, the non-parametric Kruskal-Wallis analysis can be used instead.

Basis of the calculation

The between-groups sum of squares is calculated by adding together the values obtained for each group by squaring the difference between the group mean and the overall mean and multiplying it by the number of observations in that group; that sum divided by one less than the number of groups gives the between-groups variance (or 'mean square'). The within-groups sum of squares is determined by adding together the squares of all the differences from the means in each of the groups; that sum divided by the number of observations less the number of groups gives the within-group variance (or 'mean square'). The analysis of variance is completed by dividing the between-groups variance by the within-groups variance to calculate F.

Interpretation

The probability that the group means would be observed in samples from the same population is derived from F. If the probability is not given by the computer program, a table of the distribution of F can be entered with its value and with degrees of freedom one less than the number of groups and one less than the number of observations. (If there are only two groups, analysis of variance gives the same probability value as the t-test.)

Figure 2.5   One-way analysis of variance

The weakness of analysis of variance is that even though it is a parametric test it provides only the probability that a difference exists. It does not identify, for example, a specific group whose mean differs from all the others. However, it does answer general questions such as whether recalibration contributes to imprecision.

Care should be taken in selecting and conducting further tests to identify and confirm the nature of the differences found, as the assumptions underpinning the secondary analysis are affected by the fact that a primary test has been carried out. In simple terms the degrees of freedom are reduced since the data under analysis has been constrained relative to the original experimental situation. Several of the *post hoc* tests for multiple comparisons that are available are discussed by Altman (1991) in *Practical Statistics for Medical Research.*

WITHIN-DAY AND BETWEEN-DAY IMPRECISION

Analytical variation is clinically important because it is a component of the variation that may be observed between samples from a patient taken on different occasions. Questions about the significance of observed differences in measured values are most commonly asked either of specimens taken on the same day, for example, during a metabolic function test, or of specimens taken on successive days when a patient's condition is being monitored. For these reasons it has become usual to assess both the 'within-day' and the 'between-day' analytical imprecision. 'Between-batch' imprecision becomes the only available measure when batches are run less frequently than once a day. The total SD over many weeks is of interest only because of the contribution it makes to the width of reference ranges which need to encompass the whole range of analytical variation.

In 1992 the American National Committee for Clinical Laboratory Standards (NCCLS) proposed a protocol for evaluating the precision performance of Clinical Chemistry devices. Not unreasonably it includes general guidelines about allowing sufficient time for familiarisation with a new apparatus or operating procedure, and for familiarisation with the evaluation procedure itself. It is recommended that each level of the material that is to be evaluated, preferably high, medium and low values in clinical terms, should be analysed twice within each batch of patients' specimens, and that this procedure should be repeated for twenty or thirty days. Common sense suggests that the paired analyses should be made at random within runs of patients' samples. To assess within-day imprecision when only a single batch is run each day, the specimens should be analysed near the beginning and end of the batch; if more than one batch is run the specimens should be analysed in different batches. Examination of Normal probability plots of the differences between duplicates and of the daily means will reveal any possible outliers (page 11) and will also allow the assumption of Normality to be examined. Within-day SD for each of the materials analysed is calculated from the paired analyses.

The SD of the within-batch duplicate measurements in the NCCLS protocol is independent of differences between the means of the duplicates from batch to batch or from day to day. The within-day CV can be calculated by expressing the SD as a percentage of the mean of all the measurements. The between-day SD is the SD of the means of the daily duplicates calculated in the usual way. It is thus independent of the magnitude of the differences between the duplicates.

SD FROM DUPLICATE MEASUREMENTS

Application

The calculation of SD from duplicate measurements made on a number of different subjects or materials is used to determine the reproducibility of the measurement as an alternative to making a large number of observations on a single subject or material to calculate SD directly.

Requirements

The assumption of the calculation is that the duplicates measurements are samples from populations with the same variance but not necessarily the same mean. They should, however, have mean values that do not differ too widely because there is commonly an association between mean and variance (page 9). The differences should have a reasonably Normal distribution when inspected as a Normal probability plot (page 11).

Basis of the calculation

The variance is calculated as the sum of the squares of the differences between the duplicates divided by twice the number of pairs, and the SD is its square root. The calculation is rarely available as a computer program but is readily carried out in a spreadsheet such as Microsoft Excel.

Figure 2.6 SD from duplicate measurements

The calculation of SD from duplicate measurements is useful for determining the imprecision of measurements for which no suitable control material is available. Patients specimens are used instead. Because imprecision may differ at different measured values, clinical samples that have had a single measurement made are selected to cover, for example, low, medium and high values and are then reanalysed in random order. Material of limited stability can be reanalysed the same day to calculate within-day imprecision while more stable material can also be reanalysed the following day to calculate between-day imprecision.

HOW IS BIAS ASSESSED?

Bias was defined above as the difference between the mean of a series of measurements of the same material and the true value. (In the unusual event that the error distribution of a method is logarithmic, the geometric mean, which is the antilogarithm of the mean of the logarithms of the values, is used.) Unfortunately, in laboratory practice it is rarely possible to know the true value of a biological material with any certainty. Three approaches are used:

1. A value is assigned to a material using a reference method within the laboratory. The bias of an automated haematology analyser can be assessed against values assigned to the counts of different cells in a sample of whole blood by measurement in the laboratory using manual counting chambers. Many enzyme units are defined by a rate of change under standard conditions of measurement that it is possible to repeat in the laboratory using a suitable recording spectrophotometer (as long as such factors as wave length settings, optical path cleanliness and thermostat accuracy have been checked).

2. A material is purchased with a value assigned by the manufacturer using a reference method. International and national bodies have agreed defined reference methods and primary and secondary standards for a number of assays in medical biochemistry, haematology and immunology. The use of commercially available 'quality control' materials which refer back to these primary standards is the most acceptable way of determining bias when within-laboratory assignment is not possible.

3. The mean of the values assayed in the material by the participants in an external quality assurance scheme is used. This is the least satisfactory way to determine bias because there is no absolute reference point, and because there is the danger of a drift with time should laboratories adjust their standardisation to conform with consensus values. Nevertheless, the returns from external quality assurance schemes may provide the first warning that a bias problem has developed.

Whichever material is used to assess bias, it is an advantage to examine levels that are high and low in clinical terms. An assessment of bias can be carried out at the same time that imprecision is examined using the NCCLS protocol (see Further Reading). The whole of the data at each level is first examined as a histogram or preferably as a Normal probability plot to ensure that it has a Normal distribution and to detect outliers (page 11). The next step is to carry out a one-sample t-test at each level against the assigned value. Before discussing how this is done, we will describe the t distribution.

THE *t* DISTRIBUTION

The *t* distribution was described by W S Gossett in 1908 writing under the pen-name 'Student'. For this reason the distribution is sometimes known as Student's *t* distribution and the test as Student's *t*-test. During discussion of the advantages of parametric tests in Chapter 1, it was pointed out that a single set of data is an imprecise estimate of the larger population of which it is a sample, and that all calculated values based on the sample have their own inherent imprecision. If a number of samples are taken their means are distributed about the true mean of the population. The variance of the mean of a sample is the variance of the sample divided by the number of observations; the SD of the mean is therefore the SD of the sample divided by the square root of the number of observations. To distinguish the SD of the sample from the SD of the mean, it is usual to refer to the SD of the mean as its standard error (abbreviated SE or SEM). The SE is thus smaller the larger the number of individual observations in the sample from the population, and the observed mean therefore has a narrower confidence interval.

The means of large samples from a Normal distribution which have more than 60 or so observations may be considered to be Normally distributed themselves. For smaller numbers Student proposed a similar but flatter distribution which became flatter as numbers decreased, the *t* distribution. In a true Normal distribution the proportion of observations falling within multiples of SDs from the mean can be predicted (page 10). In the same way, in a *t* distribution the probability of the true mean falling within multiples of SEs from the observed mean can be calculated. The exact shape of the distribution is determined by the 'degrees of freedom'; for a single sample this is one less than the number of observations. Degrees of freedom are so called because all but one of the deviations from the mean are independent of each other - the last can be calculated because their total must equal zero. The following Figure illustrates how the 95% confidence interval of the mean changes with degrees of freedom as the *t* distribution becomes flatter and wider.

Degrees of freedom	Number of SEs to add and subtract for 95% confidence interval of the mean
120	1.980
60	2.000
30	2.042
20	2.086
15	2.131
10	2.228

Figure 2.7 Limited table of the *t* distribution

t-TESTS

In all *t*-tests the value of *t* is calculated by dividing the quantity to be examined by its SE. The null hypothesis is that the quantity being examined does not differ from zero. The probability of the *t* value is determined from a *t* distribution with the appropriate number of degrees of freedom. The two-sample *t*-test is simply a special case of one-way analysis of variance discussed previously (page 33). However, while the latter provides only a probability value, the *t*-test has the advantage that its results can provide not only the mean difference but also the confidence interval of that difference in measurement units.

ONE SAMPLE *t*-TEST

Application

A one-sample *t*-test is applied to a single sample to test the null hypothesis that its mean does not differ from a specified value.

Requirements

The group of observations should have a reasonably Normal distribution. This can be tested by inspecting a Normal probability plot (page 11). If it does not, logarithmic transformation should be considered (page 16).

Basis of the calculation

The procedure is simply to divide the difference between the mean and the specified value by the SE of the mean to obtain a *t*-value.

Interpretation

If the probability value is not provided by a computer program, it can be read from tables of the *t* distribution entered with degrees of freedom one less than the number of observations.

The 95% confidence interval of the difference is the mean difference plus and minus its SE multiplied by 1.96 if there are more than 60 or so observations. If there are less, the multiplication factor can be read from the two-sided 0.05 probability column in a table of the *t*-distribution entered with degrees of freedom one less than the number of observations (see limited table above).

Figure 2.8 One sample *t*-test

Because, when comparing the means of control materials with their assigned values we are equally interested in positive and negative biases, a two-tailed test is used. If there is no evidence of a difference at any concentration, no bias has been detected. There are two common types of bias that might be found. In the first, absolute bias, the significant difference between the mean and the assigned value is similar at all concentrations. In the second, proportional bias, the differences differ at different concentrations, usually increasing with concentration. A combination of the two is, of course, possible. Absolute bias may result from, for example, a blanking problem while proportional bias in a method with single point calibration may indicate an incorrectly assigned value for the standard.

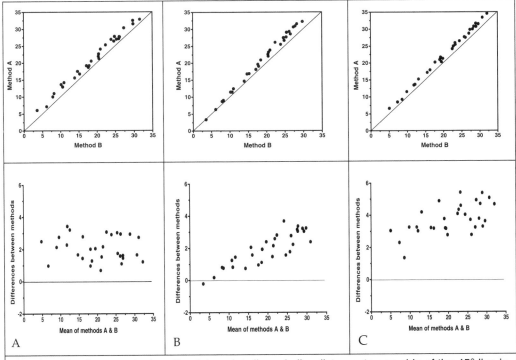

Absolute bias is present when the data points lie a similar distance to one side of the 45° line in a conventional plot and a similar distance above or below the horizontal zero difference line in an Altman and Bland plot, A. Proportional bias is present when the distance of the data points from the 45° line increases with measured value but would be negligible at zero, B. Combined bias is present when the data points diverge increasingly from the 45° line but indicate a measurable value on one axis when the other is zero, C.

Figure 2.9   Absolute, proportional and combined bias

A two-sample *t*-test can be used to test formally whether an observed bias is absolute. The null hypothesis would be that the differences between the highest mean and its assigned value and between the lowest mean and its assigned value are the same. The two groups of data to be examined are the differences between each measurement of the high material and its assigned value and the difference between each measurement of the low material and its assigned value. If data from a wide range of materials with assigned values are available, an alternative approach is to use least squares linear regression (page 52).

TWO-SAMPLE *t*-TEST: LARGE SAMPLES

Application

The two-sample *t*-test for large samples is used to test the null hypothesis that two means do not differ.

Requirements

If the samples are sufficiently large, the Central Limit Theorem states that the distribution of the sample means will be nearly Normal whatever the distribution of the observations themselves. Thus, there is no requirement for the samples to have Normal distributions. The number of observations required for the theorem to hold increases the greater the departure of the distribution of the observations from Normal. For most biological measurements, 40 to 60 observations in each sample are almost always adequate and as few as 20 may be satisfactory. There is no requirement for the sample variances to be equal.

Basis of the calculation

The SE of the difference between the means is the square root of the sum of the variances of the two sample means (SE^2). The SE is divided into the difference between the means to obtain the value of *t*.

Interpretation

If the probability that the means do not differ is not provided by a computer program, it can be read from tables of the *t* distribution entered with degrees of freedom two less than the total number of observations. The 95% confidence interval of the difference is the mean difference plus and minus its SE multiplied by 1.96 if there are more than 60 or so observations in all. If there are less, the multiplication factor can be read from the 0.05 probability column in a table of the *t*-distribution entered with degrees of freedom two less than the total number of observations in both groups (see limited table above).

Figure 2.10 Two-sample *t*-test: large samples

TWO-SAMPLE *t*-TEST: SMALL SAMPLES

Application

The two-sample *t*-test is used to test the null hypothesis that two means do not differ.

Requirements

Both samples should have reasonably Normal distributions. This can be tested by inspecting Normal probability plots (page 11). If they deviate from Normality, logarithmic transformation should be considered (page 16). In addition, their variances should not differ. This can be tested using the *F*-test (page 31). If the variances do differ, the Welch approximation can be used (see below). Alternatively, the non-parametric Mann-Whitney *U*-test can be used (page 8).

Basis of the calculation

The SE of the difference between the means of the two groups is the square root of the common variance. The latter is calculated by adding together the sum of the squares of the differences between the values and the means in each sample and dividing by two less than the total number of observations in the two groups. *t* is calculated by dividing the quantity to be tested, the difference between the two means, by its SE.

Interpretation

This is the same as for the *t*-test for large samples.

Should the variances differ, the Welch approximation calculates the probability from *t* using a reduced number of degrees of freedom. This test is provided by some computer programs. Otherwise *t* must be calculated as above and the degrees of freedom determined as follows. If SEM_1 and SEM_2 are the SEMs of the two samples and n_1 and n_2 are the numbers of observations in each, the degrees of freedom

$$df = [(SEM_1^2 + SEM_2^2)^2 / \{SEM_1^4/(n_1 + 1) + SEM_2^4/(n_2 + 1)\}] - 2$$

The result is rarely a whole number and should be rounded down.

Figure 2.11   Two-sample *t*-test: small samples

HOW IS THE DETECTION LIMIT DETERMINED?

The detection limit is defined as the smallest value that can be distinguished from zero with a defined degree of confidence. It is not possible by analysis to conclude that a substance is completely absent from a sample. For this reason it is usual to determine the detection limit by extrapolating the imprecision measured at a very low concentration to zero.

A simple approach is to choose a sample which has as low a value as possible but which gives replicate measurements that can all be clearly read. The mean and SD of the replicates are calculated. Because 95.5% of the values of a Normal distribution lie within plus and minus two SDs of the mean, only 2.25% of measurements would lie more than two SDs *below* the mean. Thus, a concentration two SDs above zero would be measurable with a probability of 97.75%. Any other probability value could be chosen in the same way. Since 10% of values lie outside the mean plus and minus 1.65 SDs, and therefore 5% lie below the mean minus 1.65 SDs, a value 1.65 SDs above zero would be detected with a 95% probability. If less than, say, 40 replicates have been measured, one should look up a table of *t* under degrees of freedom one less than the number of observations and under twice the desired probability to determine the appropriate number of SDs above zero in an analogous way. More complex approaches are discussed by Armbruster *et al* and Brown *et al* (see Further Reading).

HOW IS ANALYTICAL QUALITY ASSURED?

Quality assurance is not limited to the analytical process. It ensures the efficiency of the whole of laboratory operation, from the clinical request through obtaining, transporting, recording, storing and analysing specimens to communication of results. It includes the provision of clinical advice and also staff welfare and working conditions. It thus includes such management techniques as Total Quality Management (TQM) and Continuous Quality Improvement (CQI). In this section the rather narrower analytical aspects of quality assurance are considered.

WHY AND HOW ARE ANALYTICAL GOALS DETERMINED?

At first sight there seems little reason to set up analytical goals because all reasonable clinical laboratories will strive to achieve the lowest possible imprecision and bias. Two examples will illustrate situations where goals are needed. First, a new hormone assay has been carried out in duplicate and the means reported as recommended by the original authors of the method and by the manufacturers of the reagent kit. Is the increase in imprecision that would result from making only single measurements to save money permissible? Second, a faster and cheaper alternative to a routine method has been devised for emergency use. Is its somewhat greater imprecision acceptable? Clearly standards are required in both of these situations.

A number of approaches to goal-setting have been suggested. These have included defining allowable error as a fraction of the reference range, using the views of clinicians and laboratory workers to define a 'medically significant' CV for each test or other forms of definition by consensus about what is achievable. Criteria which are gaining increasing acceptance in Europe are based on biological variation.

REFERENCE RANGE-BASED GOALS

The most widely used approach which is based on the reference range is that proposed by Tonks in 1963. He proposed that the analytical CV should not exceed one eighth of the width of the reference range expressed as a percentage of the mean of that range. This method has the advantage that reference data are available for all clinical laboratory measurements. It has the disadvantage that the width of the reference interval itself depends on the analytical imprecision with which it was determined. A further minor disadvantage is that reference intervals often vary with age and sex.

For bias, it has been suggested that the maximum deviation from the true value should not exceed one sixteenth of the appropriate reference range or therapeutic interval if data on biological variation are not available.

CLINICALLY-BASED GOALS FOR IMPRECISION

Campbell and Owen in 1967 were the first to report the views of a number of hospital clinicians who were asked to indicate, for a small number of biochemical tests, what they considered to be acceptable analytical limits. Several similar clinical studies have been published subsequently, some incorporating the views of laboratory workers. This approach has the disadvantage that the views of end users of laboratory data are likely to be coloured by the variability of results to which they have been exposed in clinical practice. In addition, it has been shown that their opinions vary substantially with the length of their clinical experience. However, perhaps the most important difficulty is that clinical staff have no information to allow them to separate the variability of laboratory results on a patient into that part due to inherent 'biological' variability, that due to pre-analytical factors like postural change and that due to true analytical variability.

BIOLOGICAL VARIATION-BASED GOALS

A working group of the European Group for the Evaluation of Reagents and Analytical Systems has drawn together proposals using biological variation as a basis for goal setting.

To determine the true within-person biological variation of a clinical laboratory measurement it is first necessary to minimise variability due to pre-analytical factors by rigid standardisation of the conditions under which samples are taken.

The variables that may need to be controlled include:

- time of day
- timing of food intake
- recent exercise
- stress
- posture
- venous stasis during blood sampling.

After standardisation of known pre-analytical variables, it is reasonable to assume that the two remaining components of variance in a series of measurements made on an individual are analytical variance and true within-individual biological variance. In a typical investigation, a series of blood specimens are taken at specified intervals over a specified time span from 20 or 30 individuals and plasma stored in a way that ensures stability. The specimens from each individual are then measured in duplicate in random order in a single batch. The analytical variance (SD^2) is determined from the duplicates (page 35) and the total within-person variance is calculated from one of the sets of duplicate pairs. We have noted that variances have the important property of being additive (page 31). It follows that the difference between the total within-person variance and the analytical variance is that component of variance due to true biological variation within the individual. Thus:

Within-person biological variance = within-person total variance - analytical variance

One half of the average of the within-person biological SDs for the whole group of individuals is proposed as the analytical goal for imprecision.

The group total variance is calculated from all the individual single data sets. This variance minus the overall analytical variance calculated from all the duplicates gives the group biological variance (which itself is made up of the within-individual and the between-individual biological variances). Thus:

Group biological variance = group total variance - analytical variance

One quarter of the group biological SD has been proposed as the limiting goal for bias.

These approaches to goal setting have the disadvantages that the fractions are chosen rather empirically and that the goals for some analytes cannot be achieved with existing methods and instrumentation. They can, however, provide useful targets for instrument and reagent manufacturers.

State of the art goals are widely available through external quality assessment schemes, allowing comparison of performance not only with other laboratories of similar size and workload but also with other users of the same analytical method or instrument. The information provided by external schemes is of particular value when a change of instrument or methodology is under consideration. A proposed goal when data on biological variation is not available is to match the achievement of the best 20% of laboratories.

It has been argued against state of the art goals that laboratories may take special care with external assessment scheme specimens, although this is increasingly unlikely the larger and more automated the workload. However, such undesirable practices may become more widespread with the introduction of national systems for accrediting clinical laboratories. A further disadvantage is that minimal acceptable standards are not defined, so that the questions about an acceptable reduction in performance posed at the beginning of this section cannot be answered.

HOW IS ANALYTICAL QUALITY MONITORED?
Quality control developed as a system for ensuring that the products of manufacturing processes fell within narrow tolerances, usually by measuring samples taken at intervals from the production line. The results of investigations on samples from patients produced by clinical laboratories cannot have predetermined values and limits. It is therefore necessary to ensure that the analytical process is in control by incorporating known samples within batches of patients' specimens. Clinical laboratory workers sometimes fail to make a clear distinction between two different kinds of specimen that may be measured along with patients' specimens; on the one hand, those specimens that are used to control quality and on the other, those used to assess quality.

- Quality *control* materials may or may not have ascribed values for the results of analysis, and are sometimes used to 'adjust' patients' results if, for example, there is clear evidence of linear drift during the running of a batch of analyses. In this situation, least squares regression (page 52) of analytical results against specimen position numbers in the run could be used to construct an adjustment algorithm. If measured values in the batch deviate consistently from the ascribed values, an absolute or proportional adjustment may be made to the patients' results. Relying on such adjustments to correct for problems of drift or bias is not good practice. Should this become necessary on a regular basis, it is a clear indication to examine such factors as thermostatic control and calibration.

- Quality *assessment* materials have predetermined or ascribed values and are used to assess the efficiency of the quality control process. Ideally the values should be unknown to the analysts. This is rarely possible to maintain in practice, but is of little importance with automated analytical techniques that are not susceptible to operator bias. Should patients' results be adjusted using an algorithm derived from the results of quality *control* materials, the results of quality *assessment* materials must be adjusted in exactly the same way. In the event that the values after adjustment fall outside predetermined limits, the batch is rejected and must be re-analysed.

Shewhart (Levey-Jennings) charts

Industrial process sampling measurements are often plotted on Shewhart charts. They were introduced into clinical laboratories in 1950 by Levey and Jennings. The sample mean is used as a measure of the central tendency and the Normal distribution as a model for the interval. Ideally each quality assessment material is measured repeatedly over two or three weeks at a time when the method is performing satisfactorily. The mean and SD are calculated and a chart constructed with five horizontal lines: the mean plus 2 and plus 1 SDs; the mean; and the mean minus 1 and minus 2 SDs. Results of subsequent analyses of the assessment material are plotted above the appropriate patient batch number or date. Not more than one in twenty values should fall outside the 2 SD lines. The charts allow visual recognition of sudden or gradual changes in mean value, of changing imprecision over a relatively long time scale and of outliers.

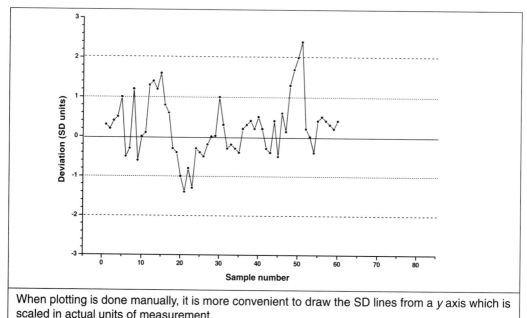

When plotting is done manually, it is more convenient to draw the SD lines from a *y* axis which is scaled in actual units of measurement.

Figure 2.12 Shewhart (Levey-Jennings) quality assessment chart

MULTI-RULE SHEWHART (WESTGARD) ASSESSMENT

Westgard and his colleagues in 1981 drew up rules based on statistical analysis of the few quality assessment results that are obtained from an individual analytical run so that an immediate decision could be made about data reporting. They recommend that analyses of two different control materials run once in each batch should be plotted on separate conventional Shewhart charts.

Briefly, if both results are within 2 SD limits, the batch of patients' results is reported. If one result exceeds a 2 SD limit, the patients' results are held and the following rules checked. The batch is rejected if:

- One result exceeds a 3 SD limit
- Both results exceed the same 2 SD limit
- Each result exceeds a different 2 SD limit
- The same material exceeds the same 2 SD limit in a previous batch
- The last four consecutive results on both materials exceed the same 1 SD limit
- The last three consecutive results on the same material exceed the same 1 SD limit
- The last ten consecutive results on both materials lie on the same side of the mean
- The last nine consecutive results on the same material lie on the same side of the mean.

This method for assessing quality before reporting is entirely compatible with the application of adjustments based on quality *control* results to both quality *assessment* specimen results and patients' results before the rules are applied. Some multi-channel biochemical analysers which include Westgard rules within their software allow this realistic approach to be used, but others do not.

CuSum CHARTS

The disadvantage of both the Shewhart chart and the Westgard's multiple rule assessment is that changes in bias may be obscured by random analytical variation. Cumulative sum (CuSum) charts originated in industrial processes where continuous inspection of deviation from a mean value was critical. As the name implies, the cumulative sum of the deviations of the measured values from the fixed mean is plotted. When the process is in control the plot is horizontal with random variations around the line of the mean, and its appearance is similar to that of a conventional Shewhart plot. However, because the plot is of cumulative values a small constant deviation of measured values from the mean results in the plot moving rapidly away from the horizontal. For example, an error of only 0.5 mmol/L in determining a mean sodium concentration will lead to an average deviation from the horizontal line of 2.0 mmol/L after only four measurements have been made even though there has been no change in bias.

A V-mask can be constructed at a horizontal lead distance from the last data point that allows control for both a defined alpha risk (suspecting that the process is out of control when it is not) and for a defined beta risk (not suspecting that the process is out of control when it is). One of those pre-defined points is reached should the CuSum plot cross one of the arms of the V. PW Strike (1991) gives full details about the construction of CuSum charts and V-masks (see Further Reading).

The CuSum plot has not been widely accepted in clinical laboratories partly because it was introduced before appropriate computer software became available, but largely because it is excessively sensitive to minor errors in determining the fixed mean.

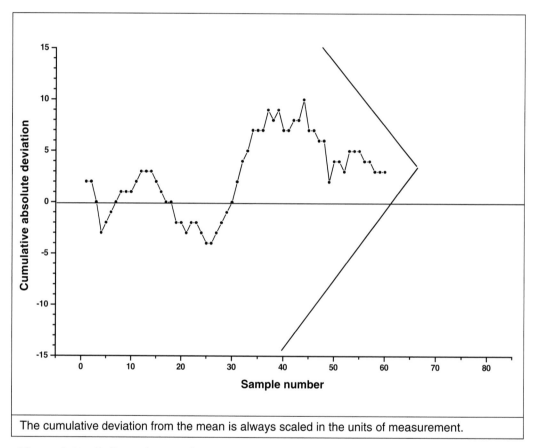

The cumulative deviation from the mean is always scaled in the units of measurement.

Figure 2.13 CuSum chart and V-mask

PATIENT MEANS

Examining patient daily means for shifts became a popular way of detecting changes in bias at the time that laboratory computers were being introduced to handle the large volumes of data produced by multichannel analysers. Before the mean for a test was calculated the whole of all patients' results that day were truncated to attempt to exclude bias caused by varying numbers of results of clinical significance, usually by using truncation limits identical with or narrower than those of the reference range. One of the difficulties was a lack of constancy in the patient population because of such factors as specialised clinics. The truncated means for urea and creatinine, for example, were always higher on renal clinic days. The introduction of discretionary analysers into clinical biochemistry has further reduced stability by removing the background of 'non-requested' results produced by non-discretionary analysers.

The method found a major place in monitoring the calibration of automated haematology analysers at a time when stable control materials were not available. More recently, stabilised cell preparations prepared from time-expired donor blood, which have a life of over six weeks, have provided a satisfactory means of detecting changes in bias. They also have the advantage of also allowing imprecision to be monitored.

DELTA CHECKS

There is no certain way to check patients' results for blunders. However, most laboratory computer systems allow a new result to be compared with the patient's most recent result. 'Surprise limits' can be defined, depending on the time interval between the results, which will alert laboratory staff to a possible problem when the limits are exceeded.

CLINICAL CONSISTENCY

The small amount of clinical information commonly provided on clinical laboratory request forms may indicate the question that the clinician is asking and the provisional diagnosis or the clinician's interpretation of a previous laboratory result. This information can prove invaluable in helping to detect blunders, such as a specimen taken from the wrong patient.

Occasionally a clinician may draw the laboratory's attention to a trend in results that has escaped the laboratory quality assurance system. Such clinical suspicions almost always have some basis in fact, though they do not necessarily result from a deterioration in laboratory performance. They always deserve thorough investigation and should never be ignored or dismissed as inconsequential.

Paradoxically, demonstrating to a clinician a rigorous approach to identifying and responding to a blunder or to a suspected deterioration in performance can increase confidence in the laboratory.

HOW ARE EXTERNAL QUALITY ASSESSMENT RESULTS USED?

External quality assessment schemes generally provide returns showing the submitting laboratory's result for each analyte together with the mean and SD of all participating laboratories' results. Specimens from external quality assurance schemes provide a retrospective assessment of performance and clearly cannot be used to control batch production. However, they can be used as an alarm system to trigger a more detailed analysis of internal quality assessment results to determine whether a deterioration in performance has been overlooked or ignored.

Schemes censor the submitted data in a variety of ways. For example, in the UK National External Quality Assurance Scheme for Clinical Chemistry, obvious outliers are first removed from the returns from all laboratories for each analyte and the remaining results are then 'trimmed' by removal of a percentage of high and low values. Trimmed means provide a robust estimate of the true means, and they are taken as consensus values. To avoid the large effect of outliers, SDs can be estimated from the trimmed samples by a method that makes mathematical allowance for the removed data.

The UK scheme provides a number of indices of performance over time. Each submitted value is expressed as a percentage difference from the consensus value. The absolute value of this percentage difference is divided by a scaling factor to provide a similar range of numerical values for each test called the Variance Index Score (VIS). The mean of the most recent 10 scores for each analyte against time is presented graphically (Mean Running VIS or MRVIS). A similar plot which combines all scores irrespective of analyte is also provided (Overall MRVIS or OMRVIS).

European schemes vary widely in the frequency and type of specimen analysed, in whether consensus means or target values are used and in their criteria for acceptable performance. In the USA proficiency testing became a legal requirement for laboratories that wanted to stay in business when the Clinical Laboratories Improvement Amendments (CLIA) were approved in 1988. However, the standards that are applied have been criticised because the way they were derived is not well documented and specimens are provided for analysis only infrequently.

HOW SHOULD AN UNACCEPTABLE EXTERNAL RESULT BE DEALT WITH?

What should be done if an external report shows that the result for an analyte differs unacceptably from the mean of all other laboratories? If the results for several analytes in the same quality assurance specimen show discrepant results, the likelihood is that the wrong specimen has been analysed or that results from a different specimen have been transcribed. If there is only a single bad result, the first action should again be to check for a possible transcription error. If the result is confirmed, it is an indication that the results of all the internal quality assessment specimens that have been analysed recently, together with results from any other external scheme, should be examined in detail for increased imprecision or bias.

Changes in imprecision and bias can be examined using data from either assayed or unassayed assessment materials. A possible deterioration could be tested formally by comparing the SDs of results for the same material over two periods using the *F*-test (page 31) and comparing the means with a two-sample *t*-test (page 40).

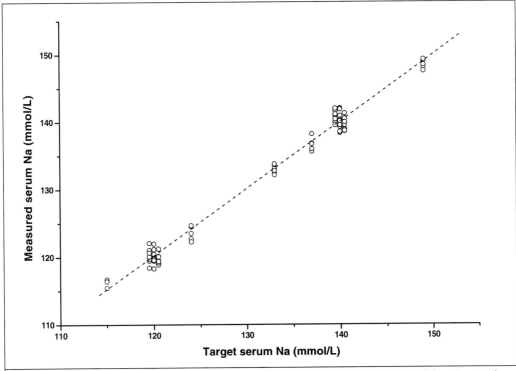

Measured results are plotted against consensus mean values, supplemented by prospective measurements of assayed control materials plotted against their assayed values. It is appropriate to use least squares linear regression for the statistical assessment of absolute and/or proportional bias because the *x* values can be regarded as having no error.

Figure 2.14 Assessment of suspected bias in external quality assurance results

If a change in mean value is identified, it may not be clear which period shows the least bias. (The external result that prompted the examination could have been an isolated blunder.) It is also important to determine whether the bias is absolute, affecting all levels of analyte equally, or proportional, showing an increasing effect with increasing level, as discussed previously (page 36). These possibilities can be explored with the recent results for assayed assessment materials and any other external scheme data that is available, perhaps supplemented with additional prospective assays to provide a wide range of measured values, by using least-squares linear regression.

LEAST-SQUARES LINEAR REGRESSION

Application

Linear regression is applied to paired measurements with the object of fitting the best straight line which will pass through the plotted points to predict the average value of one variable, the dependent variable, to be expected at any value of the other independent variable. The independent variable is usually named x and the dependent variable y. The equation of the linear regression line of y on x is usually given as $y = a + bx$; where a is the intercept on the y axis and b is the regression coefficient (slope) of y on x. An alternative nomenclature is sometimes used; $y = mx + c$

Requirements

The assumptions of least-squares linear regression are that there is a straight line which can be drawn through the means of the x and y values in such a way that the data points have a Normal distribution about it in the y direction at each value of x, and that the SDs of y are similar at all values of x. If a plot shows that this is not the case, logarithmic transformation of one or both variables should be considered (page 16). Outliers exert a disproportionate effect on the results.

Basis of the calculation

The calculation of the line of least squares is based on minimising variance in the y direction. In common with all parametric statistical tests, the calculated parameters have their own errors. Thus, the standard error (SE) of the slope defines how much the line might pivot about the central point through the means of x and y. Similarly, the SE of the intercept defines how much the line might vary in the y direction (usually plotted vertically).

Interpretation

The SEs allow calculation of the confidence intervals of the slope and of the intercept. Most statistical packages provide a probability value, the null hypothesis being that the parameters do not differ from zero. Although this may be appropriate for the intercept, it should be remembered that the relevant null hypothesis for the slope is more often that it does not differ from one. This probability can be derived from t calculated by dividing one minus the slope by the SE of the slope.

Figure 2.15   Least-squares linear regression

Quality assessment results regressed on assayed values or consensus means show absolute bias if the intercept is significantly different from zero and proportional bias if the slope is significantly different from one (Figure 2.9, page 39). A combination is, of course, possible.

HOW ARE TWO QUANTITATIVE METHODS COMPARED?

Clinical laboratory methods are compared for several reasons. The most common is that a laboratory is considering the purchase of a new analyser because an old analyser is unreliable or because the new analyser would be better able to cope with an increased workload and, perhaps, would perform analyses more economically. A second reason might be that a new method has been devised which is thought to be less imprecise, or more accurate, sensitive or specific than an existing method and a decision has to be made about whether to adopt it. A third reason might be that a quicker, more convenient or more economical adaptation has been made to an existing method which is claimed to show no deterioration in performance. In all three cases it is necessary to know whether there might be changes in imprecision or bias that would be likely to affect clinical interpretation and make it necessary to change reference ranges, action limits or therapeutic windows. If no clinically important changes are found then existing data for diagnosis can continue to be used.

Two kinds of data can be used to compare methods: either independent data about analytical imprecision, bias, specificity and working range for each method, or measurements that are made by both methods on the same clinical samples. Independent investigations are needed if formal comparisons of specificity and working range are required. However, such investigations may not be necessary in practice if the analysis of a wide range of clinical samples shows no important differences in results by the two methods. Direct method comparison is therefore usually undertaken as a first step.

The American National Committee for Clinical Laboratory Standards (NCCLS) has recommended that when comparing a new method with an existing one sufficient time must be allowed for familiarisation with new apparatus or operating procedures, just as with the formal evaluation procedure for a single method. The material used for the comparison should consist of patients' samples selected to cover the clinically encountered range of results as evenly as possible. At least sixty samples should be analysed by both methods in similarly sized small batches on the same days.

If the methods to be compared demand a high level of operator intervention, and especially if they are largely manual techniques, it is desirable that the same operators use both methods to avoid differences due to differences between operators. A particular operator-dependent problem with methods that required the manual transcription of results from, for example, a meter was digit preference – a subconscious tendency to round to whole numbers and to prefer zeros and fives. This has become unimportant in laboratory medicine with the replacement of meters by digital displays and hard-copy printouts.

There are two advantages to making duplicate rather than single measurements by each method, preferably in random order within batches:

- The differences between the duplicates within each method can be inspected for outlying values. The presence of an outlier suggests a 'processing' problem such as short sampling in one of a pair rather than an intrinsic methodological problem. If only single measurements were made, such an aberrant result might suggest a difference between the methods in specificity or in susceptibility to analytical interference.

- The analytical imprecision of each method can be determined for, say, high, medium and low values by calculating the SD by the method of duplicates (page 35). The SDs can then be compared both within and between methods using the F-test (page 31). Thus, one can determine whether the imprecision of the new method differs from that of the old and also how the imprecision of either method changes with the measured level.

A further minor advantage of duplicates is that the underlying relationship between results by the two methods can become somewhat clearer if their means rather than single values are compared because analytical noise is reduced a little.

Before statistical analysis is considered a plot of the results (or the means of duplicate results) by one method against the other should be inspected. This will allow outliers to be detected and investigated as described earlier (page 22). Interpretation is aided by including a line of equality. If the plot shows a widening scatter with higher values, then logarithmic transformation should be considered. This is particularly likely with plasma enzyme methods.

Among the tests that can be applied to describe the relationship between results by two methods are least-squares linear regression (page 52), Pearson correlation, Deming regression analysis, Passing and Bablok's method and the method of Altman and Bland. The advantages and disadvantages of each method are discussed below.

LEAST-SQUARES REGRESSION AND CORRELATION

The disadvantage of using least squares regression to describe the relation between two methods is the assumption that the independent variable is determined without error. This is a valid assumption if the question is one of prediction. For example, given an observed linear relationship between serum calcium and serum albumin concentrations, the method can be used to predict the average calcium concentration that might be expected at a specified albumin concentration. However, in method comparison one is concerned not with prediction but with description of a relationship between variables both measured with error. Neither of the slopes, x on y nor the opposite regression, that of y on x, best describes the relationship between results by the two methods. Least squares regression gives a slope that is smaller and an intercept that is greater than the true relationship, and these differences become greater the narrower the range of measured

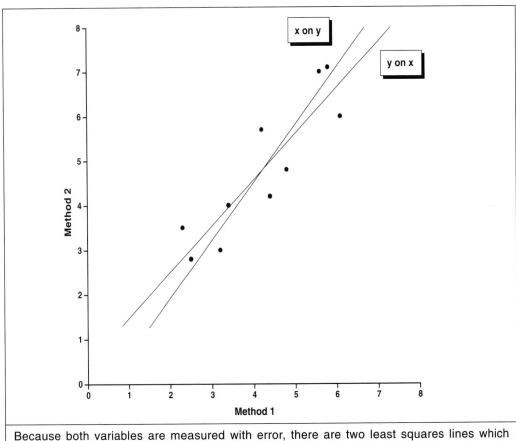

Because both variables are measured with error, there are two least squares lines which become more divergent the poorer the correlation.

Figure 2.16   Least squares regression is inappropriate for method comparison

values.

If all the points were on a single straight line, then the regression lines of x on y and of y on x would be in exactly the same position (although the regression equations would differ because one would be expressed in terms of x and the other in terms of y). If, on the other hand, x and y values were completely unrelated, the regression lines would be at right angles. Karl Pearson (1857-1936), Galton Professor of Eugenics in the University of London, introduced the correlation coefficient, r, as a numerical way of expressing how closely the slopes of the two regression lines agree. The correlation coefficient is plus one when x and y increase together on a perfect straight line, minus one when one decreases as the other increases on a straight line and zero when the lines are at right angles and there is no relation between x and y. Statistical packages give a probability for r, the null hypothesis being that there is no relationship between the variables.

The Pearson correlation coefficient gives no information of value in method comparison studies because r can be highly significant when there is an obvious bias between the two methods. An r value near one will be obtained when the data points lie close to a straight line even when the slope of the line is very different from one. It measures the strength of *association* not of *agreement*. It would, anyway, be very surprising if the probability value for r were not highly significant in a comparison of results by two methods which purport to measure the same thing.

DEMING REGRESSION

Deming adopted the approach of Kummel (1879) to solve the problem of describing the relationship between variables both measured with error by proposing that the sum of the squares of the deviations from the line should be minimised in both the x and the y directions at the same time, taking account of the analytical imprecision of each method. (Imprecision data will be available if measurements by each method are made in duplicate as recommended above.) Those without access to a computer that includes Deming's method can derive its regression coefficients from least squares regression coefficients if the imprecisions of the two methods are known (see Payne R B, 1985, Further Reading).

The major advantage of Deming's method is that it gives only a single regression line whether x or y is used as the 'independent' variable. The intercept is calculated as in conventional least squares regression as the mean of y minus the product of the slope and the mean of x or vice versa. The calculation also provides the SE of the slope and of the intercept, in the y direction if x is taken as the independent variable, so that the line can be plotted with confidence limits. (NCCLS recommend that the conventional least squares estimates of the SEs of the slope and the intercept should be used rather than the Deming estimates "because they are measured in the perpendicular direction and seriously underestimate the correct error factor"; however, no evidence for this statement is given.) The disadvantage of Deming's method is that it assumes the ratio of the analytical variances of the two methods is constant over the range of measurements. Thus, the method may be in error if the analytical SDs increase with measured values at different rates. This assumption of a constant variance ratio can be checked if duplicate measurements were made at three different levels. Like least squares linear regression, Deming's method is greatly influenced by data pairs that have substantially higher or lower values than the bulk of the results.

PASSING AND BABLOK REGRESSION

In 1983 Passing and Bablok, statisticians working for Hoechst A G and for Boehringer Mannheim GmbH respectively, published a modification of Thiel's procedure adapted to method comparison studies. Essentially, the slopes of all the straight lines between any two points are used to calculate the slope. Like Deming's method, it gives only one regression line. The method has been well publicised in the field of clinical chemistry but has not been extensively used because the method of calculation has not been widely available.

The method introduces a median shift which the authors were unable to prove theoretically was unbiased. However, one of us has validated the method by computer simulation and have shown that, unlike Deming's method, it has no bias in its estimates of slope and intercept when measurement error increases with concentration at different rates. The method has the additional advantage that each pair of results is given equal weight in the calculation so that, again unlike Deming's method, it is not unduly biased by extreme values. It has the disadvantage that it gives no measure of scatter.

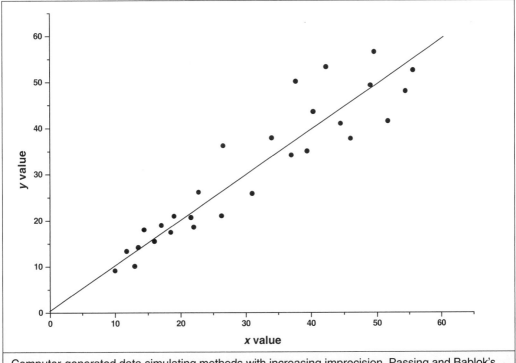

Computer-generated data simulating methods with increasing imprecision. Passing and Bablok's regression procedure is more accurate than Deming's method under these circumstances.

Figure 2.17   Method comparison when imprecision increases with value

ALTMAN AND BLAND PLOT

One way in which the agreement between two methods can be judged by eye is to draw a 45° line of equality through a plot of the points. An alternative and more informative approach was proposed in 1983 by Douglas Altman, then at the MRC Clinical Research Centre, and Martin Bland, in the Department of Clinical Epidemiology at St George's Hospital Medical School. They suggested that the differences between the methods should be plotted against the mean of the two methods. This allows one to assess visually

- the range of quantitative differences between the methods
- the presence of bias (more points above than below the horizontal zero line or vice versa)
- changes of difference with mean value
- changes of bias with mean value

Examples are given in Figure 2.9 (page 39).

If there are no changes with mean value, and the differences have a Normal distribution with no outlying values, then the mean difference and the SD of the differences can be used to calculate the confidence interval of the differences. In addition, the mean difference and its SE can be used to calculate whether it differs significantly from zero using the paired t-test.

Not infrequently methods have an increasing SD over the range of observations so that the differences between them increase with mean value. This is found, for example, with many serum enzymes. If the CVs of the methods are constant over the range, Anne Pollock and her colleagues in Manchester suggested that a plot of percentage differences against mean value could be used to display bias. If this shows a horizontal distribution of points with a constant scatter in the y direction and the differences between the percentages have a Normal distribution, the mean percentage difference and its confidence limits can be calculated. An alternative when imprecision increases exponentially with concentration is to plot the differences between the logarithms of the values against the means of the logarithms. If the differences between the logarithms show a Normal distribution, back transformation of the calculated mean and confidence limits gives the mean and the limits of the ratio of one method to the other.

Some of the difficulties that may arise with Altman and Bland difference plots have been described by Stöckl. In particular, when there is a combination of absolute and proportional bias between methods, neither a standard plot nor a percentage plot is easily described mathematically.

PAIRED *t*-TEST

Application

The paired *t*-test is applied to test the null hypothesis that the mean difference between paired observations does not differ from zero. It is therefore a special case of the one-sample *t*-test .

Requirements

The assumption of the test is that the differences between the paired observations have a reasonably Normal distribution. This can be tested by inspection of a Normal probability plot (page 11). If this assumption is not fulfilled then logarithmic transformation should be considered (page 16). The equivalent non-parametric test, Wilcoxon matched-pairs signed-ranks test, can be used if a Normal distribution cannot be achieved (page 62).

Basis of the calculation

The SE of the mean difference is calculated and the value of *t* obtained by dividing the mean difference by its SE. The degrees of freedom are one less than the number of pairs.

Interpretation

If the probability value is not provided by a computer program, it can be read from tables of the *t* distribution entered with degrees of freedom one less than the number of pairs. The 95% confidence interval of the difference is the mean difference plus and minus its SE multiplied by 1.96 if there are more than 60 or so pairs in all. If there are less, the multiplication factor can be read from the 0.05 probability column in a table of the *t*-distribution entered with degrees of freedom one less than the number of pairs (see limited table above).

Figure 2.18   Paired *t*-test

Altman and Bland chose to plot differences against the mean of the two methods because the true value is unknown and they considered the mean to be the best estimate. However, in clinical laboratory practice this is not always the case. The differences between one laboratory's measurements on external quality assurance specimens and the all-laboratories consensus values would best be plotted against the consensus values because the variance of the consensus values is very small. In these circumstances, absolute and proportional bias can be quantified using least squares linear regression rather than the Passing and Bablok procedure.

HOW ARE TWO QUALITATIVE METHODS COMPARED?

CLASSIFIED DATA

Occasionally the comparison of two methods which simply classify results as positive or negative may be needed. For example, if the sensitivity of a new batch of reagents for the detection of faecal occult blood were shown to differ from the old batch, calibration would need to be reassessed. McNemar's χ^2 test can be used to examine the results by the two methods on the same (well-mixed) faecal specimens.

McNEMAR'S CHI-SQUARED (χ^2) TEST

Application

McNemar's test is used for a two by two table of classified data that are paired, either classification of the same subjects or material treated in two different ways or classification of individually matched 'tests' and 'controls'. The null hypothesis is that the proportions of different outcomes obtained on the two occasions or between tests and controls do not differ. If the hypothesis were true there would be equal numbers in the two cells where the classifications were discordant, for example, those positive on the first occasion but negative on the second and *vice versa*.

Requirements

The test is not valid if the total of discordant pairs is less than ten. The alternative is to calculate exact binomial probabilities (see Kirkwood, *Essentials of Medical Statistics*).

Basis of the calculation

To calculate the paired χ^2 statistic including a continuity correction, one is subtracted from the absolute value of the difference between the numbers in the discordant classifications, the result squared and then divided by the sum of the discordant classifications.

Interpretation

To obtain the probability that the difference between the proportions would occur by chance without a computer, a table of χ^2 is entered with one degree of freedom.

Figure 2.19   McNemar's chi-squared χ^2 test

Comparison might also be required between two methods which classify results into a number of independent groups. Several automated haematology analysers are now available which provide a differential count, classifying white cells as neutrophils, lymphocytes, monocytes, eosinophils or basophils. The standard c2 test can be used to test the null hypothesis that there is no relation between rows and columns, that is, that the distribution of counts among the white cell classes by one machine is independent of the count distribution among classes by the other.

THE STANDARD CHI-SQUARED (χ^2) TEST

Application

The χ^2 test can be applied both to two by two tables of independent classified data and to tables with larger numbers of classes, for example, a three by four table, to test the null hypothesis that there is no relation between rows and columns.

Requirements

For the test to be valid, it has been suggested that 80% of the *expected* frequencies (see below) should be greater than five and none should be one or zero. For a two by two table, Fisher's exact test (page 6) can be used instead. For larger tables, classes could be combined to increase the expected frequencies.

Basis of the calculation

The first step is the calculation from row and column totals of the expected frequency in each cell if the null hypothesis were true. The expected frequencies are calculated by expressing the row totals as percentage of the total observations and then applying these percentages to the column totals (or *vice versa*). The square of the difference between the observed and expected frequency in each cell is then divided by the expected frequency. The χ^2 statistic is their sum. For two by two tables, Yates' correction is applied: the absolute value of the difference between the observed and expected frequency is reduced by 0.5 before it is squared and divided by the expected frequency.

Interpretation

To obtain the probability value without a computer, a table of χ^2 entered with degrees of freedom one less than the number of columns multiplied by one less than the number of rows.

Figure 2.20   The standard chi-squared χ^2 test

RANKED DATA

The Wilcoxon matched-pairs signed-ranks test is the non-parametric equivalent of the paired *t*-test. It can be used to compare qualitative tests that give a number of ordered classifications, for example urine dipsticks that give results as negative, +, ++, +++ or ++++ by assigning the results in each category ascending numerical values such as 1, 2, 3, 4 and 5.

WILCOXON MATCHED-PAIRS SIGNED-RANKS TEST

Application

The Wilcoxon test is applied either to paired ranked data, or to paired measured data when the differences cannot be fitted to a Normal distribution, to test the null hypothesis that the paired observations do not differ. If the observations are ranked each rank is assigned an ascending numerical value.

Requirements

There should be at least six differences that are not zero.

Basis of the calculation

The differences between pairs are calculated and given the appropriate sign. Pairs that show no difference are dropped from the analysis. The differences are ranked without respect to sign, tied differences being assigned the average of the tied ranks. The signs are then given to the ranks. The test statistic T is the smaller of the sums of the ranks with the same sign.

Interpretation

If the probability that there is no difference is not given by a computer program, for small numbers T can be entered in tables with the number of non-zero differences. If there are only six differences, they would all need to be of the same sign for $P = 0.05$. When there are more than fifteen differences that are not zero the probability can be calculated (see Siegel and Castellan (1988) *Nonparametric Statistics for the Behavioral Sciences*).

Figure 2.21   Wilcoxon matched-pairs signed-ranks test

SUMMARY

The performance of an analytical method is described by its imprecision, bias, specificity and analytical range. Imprecision may be concentration-dependent, so the levels at which it is determined must be defined. Bias can be absolute, proportional or a combination of the two. The detection limit of an analytical method can be determined by measuring its imprecision at a very low level.

For the comparison of quantitative methods, measurements should be made in duplicate. This allows the calculation of the imprecision of each method at a range of levels and the assessment of whether outliers are due to imprecision (when the duplicates are likely to differ widely) or to a difference in specificity or susceptibility to analytical interference between methods (when the duplicates are likely to give similar values). A plot of the results should be inspected and logarithmic transformation considered.

Least squares linear regression and Pearson correlation should not be used for method comparison. When analytical imprecision increases with the measured value, the regression method of Passing and Bablok is more accurate than Deming's procedure. Altman and Bland's plot can be used to decide whether calculation of the mean and confidence limits of the observed differences between methods is appropriate.

Methods which classify data as positive or negative can be compared with McNemar's chi-squared test (χ^2); those that classify into more than two groups with the standard χ^2 test; and those that give a number of ordered classifications with the Wilcoxon matched-pairs signed-ranks test.

FURTHER READING

Altman D G, Bland J M. Measurement in medicine: the analysis of method comparison studies. *Statistician* 1983; **32:** 307-17

Armbruster D A, Tillman M D, Hubbs L M. Limit of detection (LOD)/limit of quantitation (LOQ): comparison of the empirical and the statistical methods exemplified with GC MS assays of abused drugs. *Clin Chem* 1994; **40:** 1233-8

Bland J M, Altman D G. Statistical methods for assessing agreement between two methods of clinical measurement. *Lancet* 1986: **i:** 307-10

Brown E N, McDermott T J, Bloch K J, McCollom A D. Defining the smallest analyte concentration an immunoassay can measure. *Clin Chem* 1996; **42:** 893-903

Campbell D G, Owen J A. Clinical laboratory error in perspective. *Clin Biochem* 1967; **1:** 3-11

Deming W E. *Statistical Adjustment of Data.* New York: John Wiley and Sons Inc, 1938

Fraser C G, Petersen P H, Ricos C, Haeckel R. Proposed quality specifications for the imprecision and inaccuracy of analytical systems for clinical chemistry. *Eur J Clin Chem Clin Biochem* 1992; **30:** 311-7

Hollis S. Analysis of method comparison studies (editorial). *Ann Clin Biochem* 1996; **33:** 1-4

National Committee for Clinical Laboratory Standards. *Method Comparison and Bias Estimation Using Patient Samples; Tentative Guideline.* NCCLS Document EP9-T. (ISBN 1-56238-189-X). NCCLS, 771 East Lancaster Avenue, Villanova, Pennsylvania 19085 USA, 1993

National Committee for Clinical Laboratory Standards. *Evaluation of Precision Performance of Clinical Chemistry Devices - Second Edition; Tentative Guideline.* NCCLS Document EP5-T2. (ISBN 1-56238-145-8). Pennsylvania USA, 1992

Passing H, Bablok W. A new biometrical procedure for testing the equality of measurements from two different analytical methods. *J Clin Chem Clin Biochem* 1983; **21:** 709-20

Payne R B. Deming's regression analysis in method comparison studies. *Ann Clin Biochem* 1985; **22:** 430

Pollock M A, Jefferson S G, Kane J W, Lomax K, MacKinnon G, Winnard C B. Method comparison - a different approach. *Ann Clin Biochem* 1992; **29:** 556-60

Stöckl D. Beyond the myths of difference plots (letter). *Ann Clin Biochem* 1996; **33:** 575-7

Strike P W. *Statistical Methods in Laboratory Medicine.* London: Butterworth Heinemann, 1991

Tenner A R, DeToro I J. *Total Quality Management: Three Steps to Continuous Improvement.* Reading, Mass: Addison-Wesley, 1992

Tonks D B. A study of the accuracy and precision of clinical chemistry determinations in 170 Canadian laboratories. *Clin Chem* 1963; **9:** 217-33

Westgard J O, Barry P L, Hunt M R. Proposed selected method: A multi-rule Shewhart control chart for quality control in clinical chemistry. *Clin Chem* 1981; **27:** 493-501

Whitehead T P. *Quality Control in Clinical Chemistry.* New York: Wiley, 1977.

WILLIAM EDWARDS DEMING

Born Sioux City 14 October 1900. Died Washington DC 20 December 1993.

Deming was a Special Lecturer in Mathematics and Statistics at the National Bureau of Standards from 1930 to 1946 and Head of the Department of Mathematics and Statistics at the Graduate School of the United States Department of Agriculture from 1933 to 1953. He was a consultant to many large US companies, including Ford and General Motors. His ideas on quality improvement are considered to have had an enormous influence on the Japanese post-war industrial and economic recovery. The Deming Prize for quality achievements is broadcast on Japanese television at peak viewing time.

Deming's insight into quality control and quality improvement is nicely summarised by Will Hutton in his book *The State We're In* (London: Jonathan Cape, 1995): "Deming was a statistician who observed in the 1920s and 1930s that statistical techniques for ensuring quality control did not succeed in improving it. The issue was not assessing the statistical probability of faults within any given batch of products and trying to root them out, but how the quality of production could be improved over time. And for this Deming urged that workers had to be incorporated into the improvement of the production process... Workers' brains had to be enlisted in the achievement of quality as well as their hands; and they had to be incorporated into teams sharing a vision of continuous improvement."

Deming based his concepts on a statistician's understanding of the sources of variation in data, and on a manager's understanding of the beneficial effects of replacing fear and competition in the workplace with teamwork and co-operation. He was Honorary President of the non-profit-making British Deming Society which continues to propagate his ideas. At the age of 91 he gave a powerful ninety minute address to a meeting of the Society in Birmingham.

Deming was a modest, amusing and extraordinarily hard-working man who continued to write books, give seminars and address conferences into his nineties. He had a life-long love of music, of cats and of fresh tomatoes.

Chapter 3

Data for diagnosis and monitoring

INTRODUCTION

"Est modus in rebus, sunt certi denique fines,
Quos ultracitraque nequit consistere rectum."

"All things have their own measure; ultimately there are fixed limits
outside which something must be wrong."

Horace (65-8 BC)
Satires

Though the mainstay of diagnosis in clinical practice is the expert interpretation of a
clinical history and physical examination, it is often necessary to obtain supporting
evidence from clinical investigations. There are many different types of investigation, for
example in pathology, cardiology and radiology, but similar principles can be applied to
them all when considering their clinical usefulness. This section will use examples from
biochemistry to illustrate these principles and to point out how they can be applied to
gather maximum diagnostic information for clinical investigation.

Diagnostic tests may be used in a number of ways

- to screen for disease in apparently well persons
- to identify disease in sick patients
- to confirm a provisional clinical diagnosis
- to monitor a patient's response to treatment

The performance characteristics required of tests used in each of these situations are
different. A first line screening test should be maximally *sensitive* - that is, it should detect
all disease positive cases and should give no false negatives. On the other hand, a test
used to confirm a diagnosis should be maximally *specific* - it should not misclassify
patients as positives when they do not have the disease. A test used for monitoring needs
to be highly reproducible if changes due to treatment or disease progression are to be
detected reliably. Many tests are optimised for a particular application and sometimes
the same test may be optimised in entirely different ways to work in different clinical
circumstances.

HOW IS ABNORMALITY RECOGNISED?

There is a saying in medicine that one learns to recognise abnormal signs by observing many patients with normal features. The latter group provides a reference set against which the case in question can be compared. If a mismatch is present then it may be considered abnormal. Clinical investigations are classified using an analogous method, each test being compared against a *reference range* which describes the findings in a *reference population*. This range is sometimes erroneously referred to as the 'Normal range' which gives the misleading impression that it has a Normal distribution which in some cases it has not.

Test	Result	Reference range	Classification
Glucose - random	8.0	4.0 - 11.0 mmol/L	Normal
Glucose - fasting	8.0	3.0 - 6.7 mmol/L	Abnormal
Cortisol - 0900h	50	140 - 690 nmol/L	Abnormal
Cortisol - 12 midnight	50	<100 nmol/L	Normal
Plasma creatine kinase	800	50-140 IU/L	Abnormal
Peak flow	150	250-300 L/min	Abnormal

Figure 3.1   Some examples of reference ranges

HOW IS A REFERENCE POPULATION SELECTED?

The first step is to define the particular situation in which the reference range will be used. This is analogous to setting up the research hypothesis for a scientific experiment, the reference range effectively representing the conditions for the experimental control. To do this successfully demands a clear understanding of both the diagnostic process, the pathophysiology of the condition and the biology of the variable under investigation.

To illustrate this, consider the reference ranges for plasma cortisol in Figure 3.1. This variable shows marked diurnal variation. Collecting random samples from a group of subjects would compound diurnal variation with the random variation within and between individuals. In this case it is necessary to define representative time points, 0900h and 2400h being conventionally used, and to define reference ranges for these. Patient samples collected at these times can then be compared with the reference values to detect abnormality.

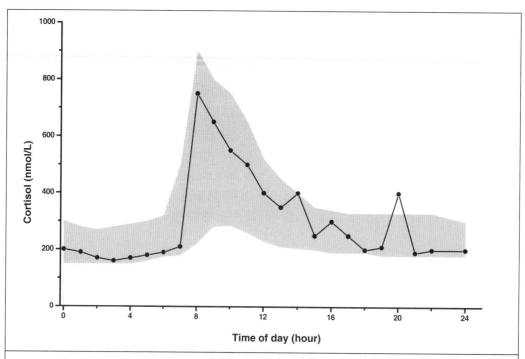

This graph shows sequential measurements of plasma cortisol in an individual patient at two-hourly intervals over the course of a day. The shaded area indicates the reference range for cortisol. Note the diurnal rhythm with higher values in the morning and the wider variation during the day than the night. The rhythm results from the variability in transient rises of cortisol due to stressful stimuli during the waking hours compared to the more stable release during sleep.

Figure 3.2   Cortisol day curve

Though the reference group may be chosen from a population representing normality, such as laboratory staff or blood donors, this is not always the case. Indeed, it is sometimes desirable to set a reference range outside that for normal individuals. It may be based on a group of patients who are chosen to be more representative of the clinical population in which we are trying to identify the diseased subgroup. For example, if we wish to diagnose patients with myocardial infarction on the basis of elevated serum cardiac markers we have several potential reference groups.

- Healthy volunteers of all ages
- Healthy volunteers of an age group who present with MI
- Hospitalised patients
- Patients presenting with chest pain who turn out after investigation not to have had an MI

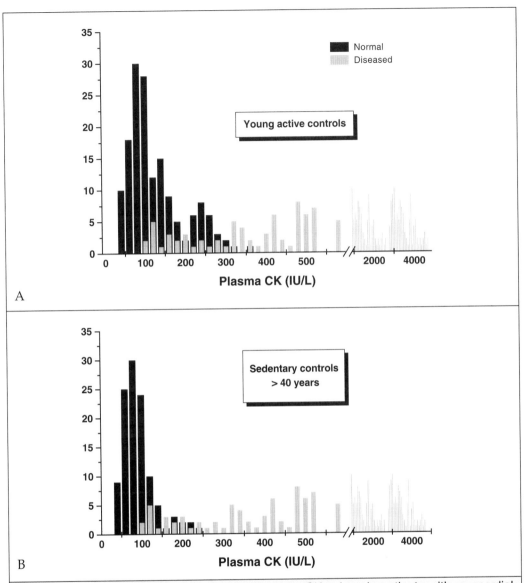

These two panels show the distributions of plasma CK values in patients with myocardial disease compared with normal subjects drawn from different sources. In A the values from young, active individuals show a bimodal distribution. In B the values for sedentary, elderly individuals show a log Normal distribution with no upper tail. Because of the lower degree of overlap between groups, better diagnostic performance would be shown by comparing patients with suspected myocardial disease with the sedentary subjects. Assuming these individuals are the population from which the patients arise, a reference range based on this group would be the more appropriate.

Figure 3.3 Creatine kinase (CK) values in young active controls compared with sedentary controls

Figure 3.3 illustrates how the contrast between the diseased and non-diseased groups may be enhanced by appropriate selection of the reference set. What is being controlled in these cases are the effects of age (plasma CK increases after puberty and falls with age) and activity (CK is higher in physically active people). Other factors such as gender (males have higher CKs) and ethnic origin (Afro-Caribbeans have higher CKs) could be similarly dealt with to produce highly specific reference ranges.

Both of these examples illustrate some of the factors which may affect the choice of a reference population and also the important corollary that the conditions of patient sampling and selection of the appropriate test can have a large influence on test usefulness.

Ideally reference ranges for measurements which are of specific diagnostic value should be determined in patients with some of the signs and symptoms of the disease being considered, but who turn out after further investigation not to have it. They form the correct control population from which the patient with the disease must be distinguished; a 'normal' reference range derived from healthy active individuals might well prove irrelevant to such patients. However, this ideal is difficult to achieve in practice, with the exception that ranges may be derived from the results of preliminary screening tests when they lead on to definitive diagnostic tests. In the future it is possible that reference ranges for diagnostic tests might be obtained if computerised data were to include provisional and final diagnoses; patients in whom these differed would be a good source of controls.

The adequacy of the concept of reference ranges depends greatly on the clinical circumstances. In many cases although reference ranges can be defined, they are redundant, either because the distinction between diseased and normal states is so marked, for example for plasma amylase in severe acute pancreatitis, or because there is such a wide degree of overlap, for example in the case of plasma urate in gout. The corresponding distributions of results from our studies are shown in Figures 3.4 and 3.5.

There are other clinical circumstances in which comparison with a reference range is inadequate for diagnostic or therapeutic purposes. For example, testing for a substance such as cholesterol, where risks of ischaemic heart disease vary continuously with plasma concentration even within the so-called normal population, requires a different approach. In this case *action limits* are defined to determine clinical decisions. Similarly, when considering the effect of drugs the concept of *therapeutic limits* is more appropriate. These concepts will be elaborated below.

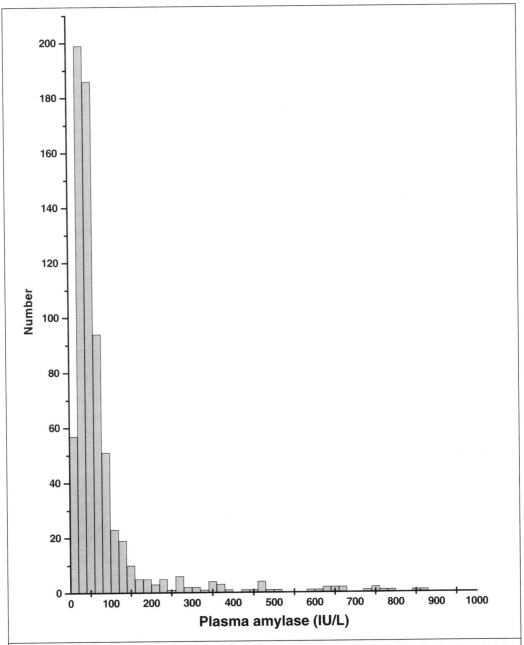

This shows the distribution of plasma amylase values obtained on laboratory specimens. Note the long right tail of this distribution. The extreme values (>800 IU/L) are from patients presenting with acute pancreatitis. The values in the intermediate range (200-700 IU/L) have been obtained from patients in the recovery phase of pancreatitis. A decision point at 2x the upper limit of normal (200 IU/L) will clearly distinguish acute pancreatitis from other conditions.

Figure 3.4 Amylase concentrations in laboratory specimens

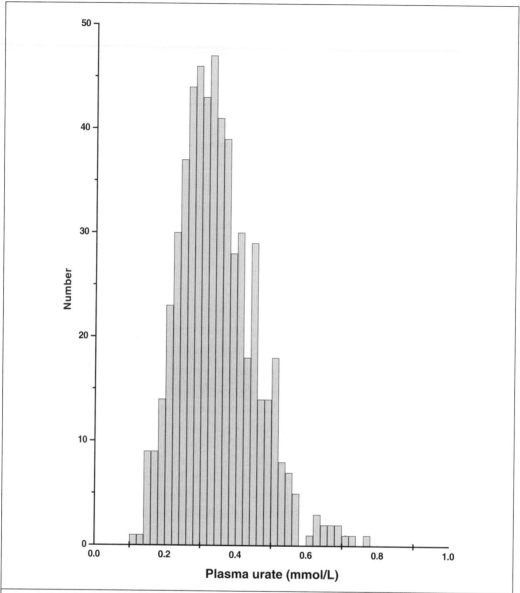

The distribution is of plasma urate values collected from the routine population screened in a local laboratory. The upper reference limit for plasma urate is approximately 0.5 mmol/L. Note the continuous nature of the urate distribution. In practice patients may develop symptoms of gout at levels of plasma urate within the reference range and conversely, many patients with levels above the reference range are asymptomatic. There is thus no clear decision point for the diagnosis of gout.

Figure 3.5   Urate concentrations in laboratory specimens

HOW ARE REFERENCE RANGES CALCULATED?

Three basic methods which can be applied to determine a reference range are :

Intuitive assessment which provides a rule of thumb guidance as to the expected upper and lower limits of a particular value.

Non-parametric methods, where cut-offs are applied manually to a set of data to determine the central 95% fraction.

The Gaussian method, where the data is fitted to a Normal distribution either directly or following transformation and the centile limits determined from parametrically derived descriptive statistics.

The International Federation of Clinical Chemistry (IFCC) has published a set of recommendations on acceptable methods for deriving reference ranges from the reference sample. The traditional method of describing a reference range is to use a range of mean + 1.96 SD which encompasses 95% of the reference sample. However, such data are not always Normal and this simple approach could produce inaccurate reference ranges leading to false classifications.

Several mathematical techniques may be utilised to establish a reference range and though statistically there may be preferences for choosing more elaborate approaches, in practice the interpercentile intervals are the most commonly used. This is because the differences between the methods are very small when based on sample sizes of a hundred or more patients and because the reference range is not a rigorous set of scientific limits. To quote the IFCC :

> *"A reference range merely serves as the basis for a more or less intuitive assessment of the biological information given by an observed value".*

Of the two approaches recommended by the IFCC, parametric methods rely on the fact that the data fit a specific distribution, usually Normal, or that with the application of an appropriate transformation the distribution may be fitted to such a curve. Non-parametric methods make no assumptions about the shape of the distribution and may be performed without elaborate computation. The IFCC favours inter-centile intervals since they are easily determined for both Normal and non-Normal distributions. The convention is that the reference interval should include the central 95% fraction of the reference distribution, although asymmetric or other fractions may be appropriate in certain circumstances as indicated below.

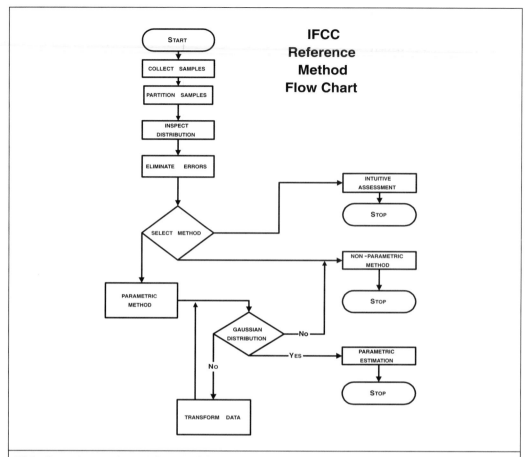

This flow chart, adapted from IFCC publications, shows the decision steps which can be followed to create a reference range. The common processes of sample collection and partitioning are followed by the selection of appropriate mathematical methods. Selection of the parametric method depends upon assessment of whether the data have a Normal distribution before or after transformation. If not, it is possible to proceed to the non-parametric method.

Figure 3.6 IFCC reference methods

The flow chart in Figure 3.6 is adapted from the procedure recommended by the IFCC for achieving a reference range. It will be noted that the stages of reference material collection are the same in all instances. Attention must be paid to controlling the conditions under which samples are collected and stored to reduce the introduction of unrepresentative variation. It should be appreciated however that collecting samples in a manner that is more fastidious than that used in routine practice could be as inappropriate as taking inadequate precautions since the reference range generated might then be somewhat artificial.

One frequently asked question is the number of reference values required. The imprecision of the method will decrease as the sample size increases. Thus, the confidence intervals which can be applied to the centile determinations will be smaller if larger numbers of values are determined for the reference set. As a rule of thumb, the minimum number of subjects should be well in excess of the number reached by dividing 100 by the lower centile limit. For 95% limits this would be 100 / 2.5, that is more than 40 subjects. This, it should be stressed, is the minimum number required. In practice, the IFCC recommends that a minimum of 120 values is used in determining a reference range. The IFCC also recommends that the confidence intervals of the centiles should be computed in order to determine whether the precision of the reference limits is sufficient for their intended use.

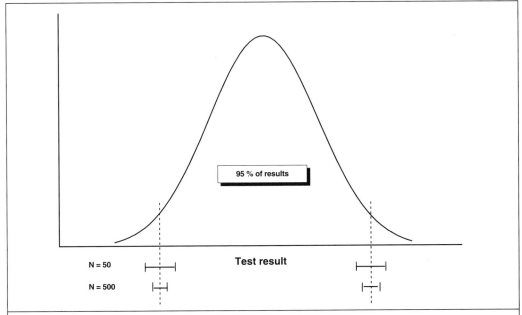

This graph illustrates diagrammatically the effect of increasing sample numbers on the confidence that can be placed on reference limits. Assuming that a parametric approach has been taken then the limits would be set to include 95% of the reference population's results. These limits are themselves subject to uncertainty and this can be reduced by increasing the size of the reference population used.

Figure 3.7 Change of confidence intervals of centile limits with numbers

It is often desirable to create reference ranges which are segregated in relation to gender or age or other such factors. This process is known as *"partitioning"*. The analysis of numbers required clearly applies to each partition so that a reference range based upon gender difference would require 120 samples from males and 120 samples from females in order to derive the appropriate limits. Clearly, age partitioning can lead to the requirement for very large numbers of samples which may not be obtainable in clinical practice. For example, obtaining large numbers of samples from normal children can be particularly difficult.

Once the data have been collected, the first recommended procedures are to inspect the distribution visually by plotting it as a histogram or a Normal probability plot, checking it for skewness, kurtosis, bimodality etc, and to consider logarithmic transformation and the exclusion of outliers as described in Chapter 1. Having inspected the data it is then necessary to choose the method for reference interval determination.

INTUITIVE ASSESSMENT

The intuitive assessment is best avoided but may be appropriate should, for example, the distribution be markedly bimodal or perhaps indicate that a particular metabolite may be undetectable under normal circumstances. Where only a very small number of values is available such as, for example, in the case of measurements in a rare disease, comparison of individual patient results against a list of values obtained in normal patients may serve a useful clinical purpose as a guide to interpretation.

THE NON-PARAMETRIC METHOD

In the absence of appropriate computing facilities, or in relatively clear cut cases, then the non-parametric method can be employed. This method requires that the data be ranked from 1 to n, the rank number of the 2.5% centile being calculated as $0.025(n+1)$ and that of the 97.5% centile as $0.975(n+1)$. The reference interval is set at the rank number equivalent to this value if the rank number is a whole number or, if the rank number is not a whole number, to a figure interpolated between the two adjacent reference results.

Confidence intervals for these values can be computed using the data in the table below which shows the rank number limits for a range of sample sizes. For the intermediate values readers are referred to the IFCC expert discussion papers.

THE PARAMETRIC METHOD

If, on inspection, the data appear to have a Normal distribution, then the centiles and their confidence intervals can be calculated using parametric statistics. In some cases it is necessary to carry out tests to confirm that data is indeed distributed in a Normal manner and the tests recommended by the IFCC include the Kolmogorov-Smirnov test and the Anderson Darling test. Should the data require transformation, the tests for a Normal distribution are applied subsequently.

Sample Size	90% CI for 2.5% centile		90% CI for 97.5% centile	
	Lower rank	Upper rank	Lower rank	Upper rank
120	1	7	114	120
200	2	10	191	199
350	3	12	239	248
300	3	13	288	298

Figure 3.8 **Confidence intervals of centiles**

The reference limits are calculated from the arithmetic mean and SD of the reference data using the appropriate standard Normal deviate value. For 2.5% and 97.5% centile limits this value is 1.96, so the SD multiplied by 1.96 is subtracted from and added to the mean to obtain the reference interval. Similarly, the SD multiplied by 1.645 subtracted from and added to the mean would provide 5% and 95% limits.

A confidence interval can be calculated for centile limits, their variance is contributed to both by the variance of the mean and the variance of the standard deviation. The 95% confidence intervals of 2.5 and 97.5% reference limits are obtained by subtracting from and adding to them the reference data standard deviation multiplied by 3.35 and divided by the square root of the number of observations. For 90% confidence intervals a multiplication factor of 2.81 is used instead of 3.35.

A WORKED EXAMPLE
Distribution of serum aspartate transaminase (AST) values in samples from 250 blood donors (125 males and 125 females), is shown in Figure 3.9 and is skewed to the right. When transformed to logarithms the data produces a distribution closer to Normal.

The distributions of the results from the male and female blood donors when shown separately were also skewed and therefore required similar transformation before analysis. The means and SDs of the log transformed values are shown in Figure 3.10. (The anti-logarithm of the log mean is sometimes called the geometric mean. Because the logarithms have Normal distributions it would be possible to use them for parametric statistical tests such as the *t*-test and the *F*-test.)

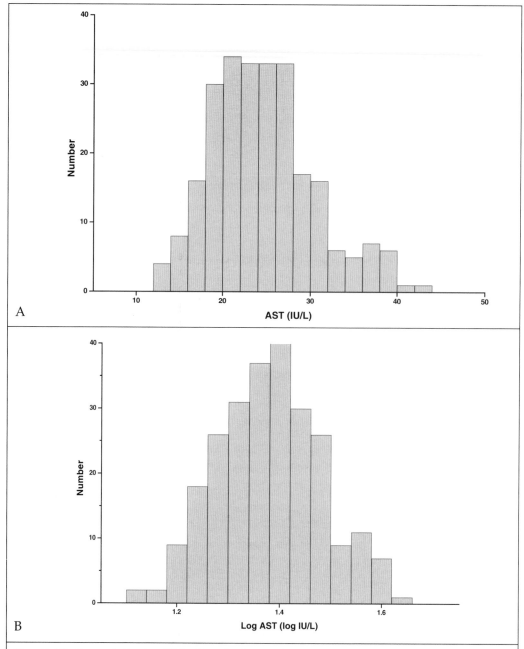

The distributions of plasma AST values in the combined population are shown before (A) and after (B) logarithmic transformation. Note that the untransformed values show marked skewness but that the transformed data are Normally distributed. The reference ranges for each of these distributions are shown in Figure 3.11.

Figures 3.9 Reference ranges for AST

Group	Number	Log mean	Log SD
Male	125	1.408	0.1006
Female	125	1.348	0.0961
All	250	1.378	0.1027

Figure 3.10 Means and SDs of AST values after logarithmic transformation

The calculated 95% reference interval for the three groups of data together with the 90% confidence intervals for the reference limits are shown in Figure 3.11.

To illustrate the mathematics, the male 95% reference limits were calculated by multiplying the log SD, 0.1006, by 1.96 and subtracting the product, 0.197, from and adding it to the log mean 1.408. The antilogarithms of the results, 1.211 and 1.605, give 16.2 and 40.3 as the 2.5% and 97.5% reference limits. The 90% confidence intervals of the reference limits were calculated by multiplying the log SD, 0.1006, by 2.81 and dividing by the square root of the number of males, 11.18. The result, 0.0253, was subtracted from and added to the logarithms of the limits, 1.211 and 1.605, and antilogarithms of these values taken to obtain the confidence intervals.

Group	Lower 2.5% limit (90% CI)	Upper 97.5% limit (90% CI)
Male	16.2 (15.3 - 17.2)	40.3 (38.0 - 42.7)
Female	14.4 (13.6 - 15.2)	34.3 (32.4 - 36.3)
All	15.0 (14.4 - 15.6)	38.0 (36.4 - 39.6)
All (non-parametric)	15 (12 - 16)	38 (36 - 40)

Figure 3.11 Calculated reference limits and their confidence intervals

Also shown in Figure 3.11 for comparison are the non-parametrically derived reference limits and confidence intervals for all the data. The results were first sorted in ascending order from 1 to 250. The 2.5 centile was 251 multiplied by 0.025, 6.3, and the 97.5 centile was 251 multiplied by 0.975, 244.7. Both the 6th and the 7th values were 15, and both the 244th and 245th values were 38, so these were taken as the reference limits. Their confidence limits were taken as the 3rd to the 12th and the 239th to the 248th results respectively (see Figure 3.8). It can be seen that the non-parametric results differ very little from those obtained by the more complicated use of transformation and parametric calculation.

HOW CAN PATIENTS PROVIDE REFERENCE DATA?

In some limited circumstances useful information can be derived from a laboratory database of patients' results, and from the prospective analysis of patients' specimens received by the laboratory.

FROM THE LABORATORY DATABASE

There are two situations where laboratory data is useful: when a test has a very low prevalence of abnormal results and when other tests can be used to eliminate likely abnormal results. In both situations minor contamination of the data is probable and a Normal probability plot of the laboratory values or the values after logarithmic transformation will usually show some deviation from linearity at one or both extremes. A 95% reference interval can be derived by drawing a straight line through the bulk of the points and reading the 2.5% and 97.5% limits from the line.

Using the laboratory database to derive or check a reference interval is particularly applicable to diseases where there is a high index of clinical suspicion, perhaps because the condition is treatable, but where there is a low prevalence in those screened. Examples include the measurement of urine catecholamine excretion in young hypertensives to exclude phaeochromocytoma, the first sweat test in children with chronic lung disease and screening tests for a variety of inborn errors of metabolism in infants.

The prevalence of abnormality can be reduced by using other database information. To derive an algorithm to adjust serum total calcium for albumin concentration it is essential to use data from patients so as to obtain a wide range of albumin concentrations, but it is also essential to minimise the number of patients who have true disturbances of calcium homeostasis. This can be achieved by excluding patients with raised urea, creatinine, transaminase or alkaline phosphatase values, those attending departments of endocrinology, haematology, oncology and nephrology and those on parenteral nutrition. Normal probability analysis of adjusted calcium values after these exclusions has shown that contamination is minimal (Barth *et al*, 1996).

BY PROSPECTIVE ANALYSIS OF LABORATORY SPECIMENS

For most tests in clinical pathology the prevalence of abnormality makes it impossible to derive reference intervals by mathematical manipulation of patients' results that have been requested by the clinician. It has been found that abnormality is much less common when specimens are analysed for tests that have *not* been requested and, not unexpectedly, that the prevalence of abnormality in non-requested analyses is lower in outpatients than in inpatients. The lowest prevalence of abnormality for biochemical tests was in patients referred to the laboratory by general practitioners for haematology investigations. Reference intervals need to be checked periodically, particularly when methods change. There was good agreement between the reference intervals from blood donors and from general practitioner haematology outpatients for urea and electrolytes, liver function tests and calcium without the need to eliminate any outpatient values by Normal probability analysis (Little *et al*, 1974).

There is difficulty in obtaining reference data for children because of the practical and ethical problems of obtaining specimens from healthy children. Specimens for this purpose, covering a wide age range and with a low prevalence of haematological and biochemical abnormalities, may be obtained from children referred to the laboratory by general practitioners for allergy investigations (IgE and RAST tests).

MULTIPLES OF THE MEDIAN - A SPECIAL TRANSFORM

In some circumstances it has proved necessary to establish reference data which is transferable across laboratories and the populations they serve because of differences between analytical techniques. It is assumed, because of the low prevalence of values that are of clinical significance in the population tested, that the median will be stable and that deviations from the median will reflect a comparable and transferable measure of individual differences from the population as a whole. The median is calculated from a pool of data generated for a particular assay and individual measured values are transformed to multiples of the median (MoMs) simply by dividing them by the median value. This transformation has been most important in screening programmes, such as those for neural tube defects and Down's syndrome which apply statistical techniques to MoMs, to assess the risk of abnormalities being present. In some cases the data is log transformed and adjusted to take into account factors such as maternal weight. The area is rather complex, involving extensive calculations of likelihood ratios (page 110) to calculate individual risks.

FAMILIAL REFERENCE RANGES

The discussion thus far has considered reference ranges in relation to the whole population at risk of disease. In many situations this can be inappropriate especially when parameters under investigation are regulated biologically within narrow ranges.

There is evidence from twin studies for the partial heritability of the serum concentrations of urea and urate, of albumin, bicarbonate, bilirubin, creatinine, globulin, phosphate and potassium and, from studies in siblings, of calcium and magnesium. In the last study variation between families was found to account for 37% of the reference interval for albumin-adjusted calcium (Payne *et al*, 1986). It would be possible for an individual's value to change by as much as 0.30 mmol/L from the family set point as the result of a significant, possibly symptomatic, disturbance of homeostasis without leaving the population reference interval of 2.20 to 2.60 mmol/L.

Familial benign hypercalcaemia - In this condition there is a genetically determined elevation in the set point of calcium required to regulate parathyroid hormone (PTH) concentrations. This leads to hypercalcaemia but without any significant consequences. Patients have normal plasma PTH concentrations and normal rates of calcium turnover and excretion, and are not at risk of renal stones, nephrocalcinosis or bone disease. The biggest danger is that they are misdiagnosed as hyperparathyroid and undergo unnecessary parathyroid surgery. The secret to the confirmation of diagnosis is to measure calcium concentrations in first degree relatives which demonstrates that the hypercalcaemia results from an inherited increased set point for calcium, an example of a familial reference range.

BIVARIATE REFERENCE RANGES INCLUDING DYNAMIC TESTS

On occasion a single univariate reference range becomes inadequate to identify abnormalities. This is especially the case for biological variables which are under homeostatic control, principally hormones, or where dynamic function tests employing physiological or pharmacological stimuli have been applied. Examples are the assessment of parathyroid hormone or insulin homeostasis. A parathyroid hormone level can rarely be interpreted in the absence of a simultaneously obtained estimate of serum calcium. This is because parathyroid hormone secretion varies with plasma ionized calcium and a high plasma concentration could be equally consistent with the presence of a parathyroid adenoma or of vitamin D deficiency, depending upon the prevailing calcium concentration. Similarly for insulin, elevated concentrations are found in insulinomas resulting in low glucose values but similar levels may be seen post-prandially in normal subjects as a consequence of an increase in plasma glucose concentration.

It is therefore valuable to display such data graphically and to consider the values in relation to the expected normal physiological response.

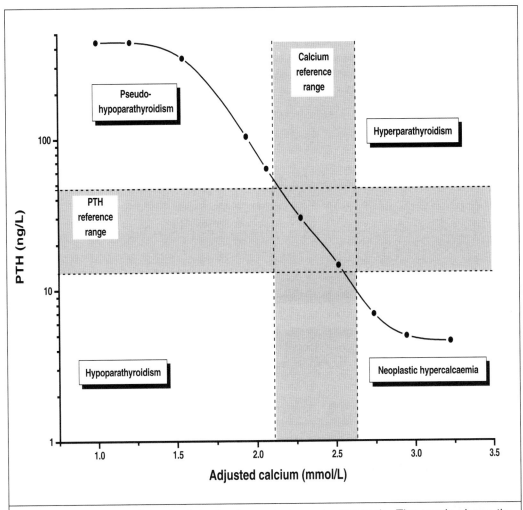

This figure illustrates the use of dual reference ranges in diagnosis. The x axis shows the albumin-adjusted serum calcium concentrations and the y axis the corresponding PTH concentrations. The line represents a normal physiological curve of control of PTH showing the negative feedback on hormone release with increasing plasma calcium. Indicated in hatched areas are the reference ranges for both calcium and PTH. Results for the majority of normal patients would lie in the central overlapping box. The figure indicates four possible diagnoses when values lie outside this box. For example, a raised calcium in the presence of a suppressed PTH level indicates that the parathyroid glands are showing normal negative feedback and thus the hypercalcaemia is likely to be the primary event, as in metastatic hypercalcaemia. In contrast, a raised calcium in the presence of a raised PTH is consistent with primary hyperparathyroidism.

Figure 3.12 Relationship between PTH and calcium concentration

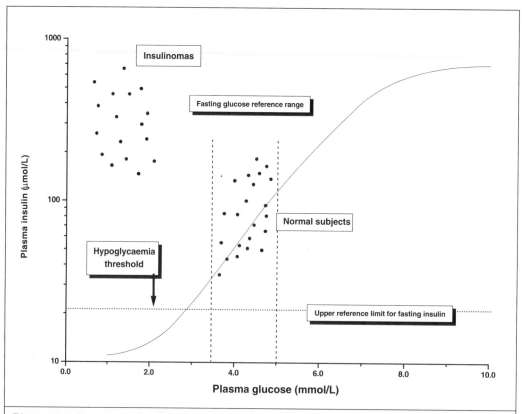

Plasma insulin values can only be interpreted with knowledge of the corresponding glucose value. The figure shows the normal relationship between plasma glucose concentration and plasma insulin concentration, plasma insulin rising as plasma glucose increases. The graph indicates that for a fasting individual an insulin of around 20 µmol/L would be expected, corresponding to a glucose value at the lower limit of normal. Also shown are representative values for normal patients and for samples from patients with insulinoma who have markedly elevated insulin values for the prevailing glucose concentration. Note that the latter insulin levels could be deemed to be normal were the prevailing glucose concentrations above 4.0 mmol/L. By combining information from both the glucose and the insulin results, it is possible to make a clear diagnosis of this rare condition.

Figure 3.13   Diagnosing insulinomas

WHAT OTHER REFERENCE VALUES ARE USED FOR DIAGNOSIS AND TREATMENT?

ACTION LIMITS

In many situations we are not so much interested in detecting abnormality as in determining whether or not to take clinical action. The risk of developing coronary heart disease is directly related to plasma cholesterol concentration and the risk is increased even at levels well inside the reference range determined by conventional methods. In this case action limits for intervention have been determined by studying epidemiological data from large populations. From these studies it is possible to determine the balance of risks of treatment and non-treatment for patients with varying concentrations of plasma cholesterol and to arrive at recommended courses of action. The influence of data from other sources such as knowledge of the patients weight, smoking history, age and family background can also be taken into account to create an overall risk assessment and interventions can be tailored for individual patients.

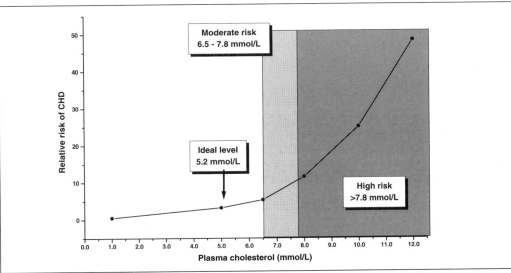

The figure shows the continuous relationship between plasma cholesterol and the relative risk of coronary heart disease. The internationally agreed degrees of risk in relation to the cholesterol value are overlaid. The consensus view is that there is an ideal maximum cholesterol level of 5.2 mmol/L which confers minimal risk. Patients with values above this but below 6.5 mmol/L are considered to be at low risk and would normally be advised to take general measures to improve their plasma cholesterol level, such as increased exercise and dietary modification. Patients with values between 6.5 and 7.8 mmol/L are considered to be at moderate risk of increased coronary heart disease so more intensive dietary measures and monitoring are usually instituted. Above 7.8 mmol/L patients are considered to be at high risk of coronary heart disease and very intensive dietary measures are usually employed. Once dietary control has been maximised it is often necessary to proceed to the use of therapeutic agents such as the statins or cholestyramine.

Figure 3.14   Action limits for cholesterol

Other examples of action limits can be drawn from the field of poisoning where limits are often applied to determine the need for the use of antidotes or other clinical interventions. Paracetamol poisoning is one common circumstance where this applies, the drug level at known time points after drug ingestion being used to trigger the use of N-acetylcysteine or methionine based on the known relationship between drug level and risk of severe hepatic damage.

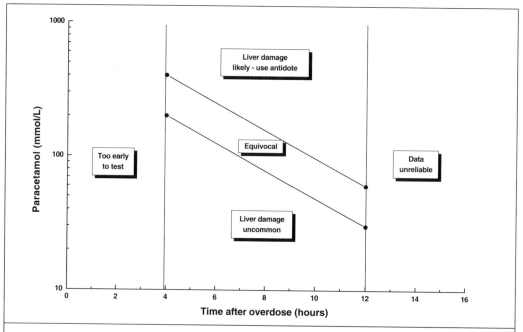

More complex action limits are used to determine the appropriate treatment for patients presenting following paracetamol overdose. The graph is based on the known relationships between paracetamol concentrations, times post-overdose and propensity to liver damage and is used to determine whether patients should receive the antidotes methionine or acetylcysteine. Note that the test is reliable only after 4 hours post-overdose and is increasingly unreliable beyond the 12 hour period. Patients with high values within the 4-12 hour window are most at risk and therefore most likely to benefit from treatment with an antidote. Patients with low levels are unlikely to suffer damage, are unlikely to benefit from treatment and indeed may be at risk from associated from side-effects and idiosyncratic reactions.

Figure 3.15 Action limits for paracetamol poisoning

THERAPEUTIC RANGES

Reference ranges for drugs are based, not on conventional ranges, but on upper and lower therapeutic concentrations. The former is set at the maximum concentration allowable without significant risk of side effects and the latter at the minimal effective plasma concentration. This range provides the therapeutic window. The exact values for these limits are seldom subject to the same rigorous analysis as that used to define reference ranges. They err on the side of safety and should not be considered prescriptive. In the final analysis they provide guides for clinical use and the best approach will be to ensure that the patients outcome is optimal with minimisation of symptoms and avoidance of side effects. This may require that patients be maintained persistently with high or low blood concentrations. For a fuller discussion, see the book in the Clinical Biochemistry in Medicine series on Therapeutic Drug Monitoring.

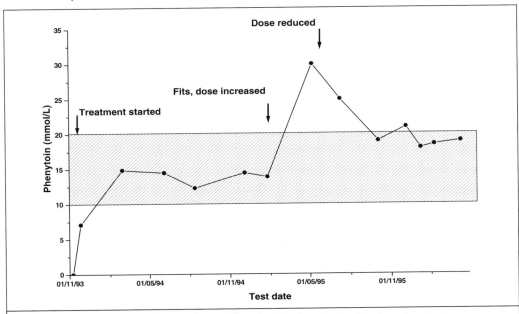

This figure shows results of plasma phenytoin estimations in a patient taken over a two year period. It shows that several weeks passed before therapeutic dose levels were achieved. During late 1994 the patient suffered from a loss of control of fits and consequently drug dosage was increased. On the following occasion the patient was noted to have symptoms of toxicity confirmed by a high plasma phenytoin level. When the dose was reduced to an intermediate value plasma concentrations fell to the upper limit of the therapeutic range and the patient remained symptom-free. There is a need to monitor the levels of certain drugs with narrow therapeutic windows and on occasion to individualise dose levels even within the therapeutic range.

Figure 3.16 Therapeutic drug monitoring

Where possible it is better that a biological outcome parameter is used for therapeutic monitoring rather than raw drug concentrations which often have no relation to efficacy. A good example is dosing for warfarin where the controlling variable is the plasma International Normalised Ratio (INR) of the prothrombin time which is treated as a therapeutic target range defined by a balance of risk and benefit.

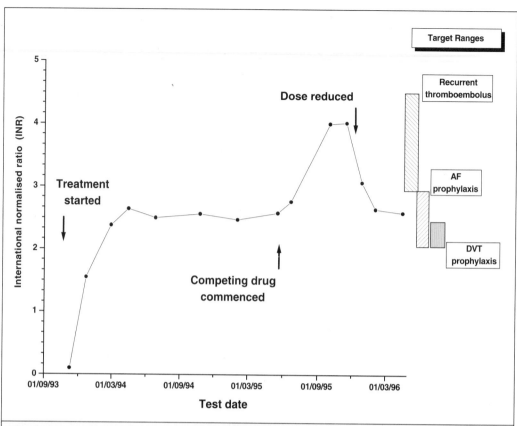

The figure shows the plasma International Normalised Ratio (INR) values of a patient treated with warfarin for prophylaxis against thromboembolism in atrial fibrillation (AF). The therapeutic range was reached relatively quickly but, following the introduction of anticonvulsant therapy, which can enhance the action of warfarin, the INR rose to values inappropriate for the clinical condition. Following dose reduction the INR fell but had not reached the appropriate level by the end of the treatment period under review.

Figure 3.17   Controlling anticoagulants

In this section we have discussed the various techniques for defining limits that can distinguish normal from abnormal, and the use of action limits and therapeutic ranges. The following section will provide an overview of how it can be shown that these limits are actually performing adequately in clinical practice. Though they may work theoretically, which techniques can be employed to assess overall performance when they are applied to the clinical population?

HOW IS DIAGNOSTIC PERFORMANCE DEFINED?

In this section we will describe a number of measures which can be used to define test performance. Through a number of illustrative cases we will explore the strengths and weaknesses of using these measures to optimise test performance.

WHY ATTEMPT TO DESCRIBE THE PERFORMANCE CHARACTERISTICS OF A DIAGNOSTIC TEST?

Evidence provided by an investigation has to be understood in combination with other sources of clinical information. Tests are rarely definitive. If they were, then it follows that large areas of clinical practice would be rendered obsolete. In order to be able to weigh test effectiveness, test performance must be described in terms which allow objective judgements to be made. It is necessary to compare tests, for example, when choosing which of two similar tests to include in a laboratory repertoire. Similarly, tests form part of an overall clinical decision process and objective methods are needed to be able to assess test performance in relation to the other sources of evidence contributing to the clinical decision.

This is not necessarily as simple as it sounds. Test performance is often dependent upon clinical circumstances and, depending on the diagnostic problem, one test may prove valuable in one situation and useless in another. Therefore, as well as understanding the measures which can be used, it is also important to appreciate the manner in which they should be used.

SENSITIVITY AND SPECIFICITY

The performance of diagnostic tests is usually described in terms of *sensitivity* and *specificity* which are defined in Figure 3.18.

Sensitivity	Proportion of patients with the disease who are correctly identified by the test	$\dfrac{\text{True positive tests}}{\text{Total patients with the disease}}$
Specificity	Proportion of patients without the disease who are correctly identified by the test	$\dfrac{\text{True negative tests}}{\text{Total patients without the disease}}$

Figure 3.18 Definitions of test sensitivity and specificity

Ideally a test should be 100% sensitive and 100% specific, that is a test which is never wrong. Unfortunately it is rare that such a test is found as the values for a variable in healthy and diseased groups generally show a degree of overlap. Thus sensitivities and specificities are often well below 100%.

A further problem which can cause over-estimation of the performance of diagnostic tests is the failure to deal adequately with information from equivocal test results. This has been highlighted by Garcia-Romero and colleagues in a letter to the Lancet in 1996. They suggest that where results are equivocal the patients data should still be included in the calculations as their omission introduces bias.

Thus, 'Total patients with the disease' should be made up of 'True positive results + False negative results + uncertain results in those with the disease', and 'Total patients without the disease' should be made up of 'True negative results + False positive results + uncertain results in those without the disease'.

PREDICTIVE POWER, POSITIVE AND NEGATIVE

Whereas sensitivity and specificity define the performance of a test in terms of the samples under test it is more common to wish to know how to interpret the value of a test in an individual case. The characteristic of predictive power is helpful here as it transforms the results of a test into the probability that the patient does or does not have the disease in question.

Positive predictive value	Proportion of patients with a positive test who are correctly diagnosed as disease positive	$\dfrac{\text{True positive patients}}{\text{Total positive tests}}$
Negative predictive value	Proportion of patients with a negative test who are correctly diagnosed as being disease free	$\dfrac{\text{True negative patients}}{\text{Total negative tests}}$

Figure 3.19 Definitions of positive and negative predictive value

The positive predictive value can be directly interpreted as the probability that a patient has the disease given a positive test. Conversely for a negative result, the negative predictive value is the probability that the patient is truly disease free.

It is incorrect to assume that tests with high sensitivity will always have high positive predictive power or that those with high specificity will have high negative predictive value. Sometimes, in order to gain high sensitivity, many false positives may have to be generated. To obtain high specificity the price may be to accept a high rate of false negative results. High numbers of false positives or false negatives will lead to lower predictive values as they reduce the proportion of true results.

EFFICIENCY

A final value which is sometimes quoted is the *efficiency* of a test procedure.

Efficiency	Proportion of patients correctly categorised	$\dfrac{\text{True negative + true positives}}{\text{Total patients tested}}$

Figure 3.20 Definition of test efficiency

Though easily calculated the value of the calculation is dubious as similar efficiencies can be obtained from tests with widely varying features. It is always preferable to consider the detailed test characteristics of sensitivity, specificity and predictive values directly in relation to the circumstances of the application of the test and the desired outcome.

THE EFFECT OF PREVALENCE

An extremely important factor that cannot be overemphasised is that the values for positive and negative predictive value are critically dependent upon the prevalence of the abnormal condition within the total population tested. In Figure 3.21 we have shown examples of the application of a test with identical upper limits set at the upper reference value tested against several experimentally-derived samples of abnormal patients with identical means and SDs. The reference population has a mean of 100 units and SD of 25 units giving an upper 95% reference limit of 150 units. The populations of abnormal patients all have a mean of 165 units and an SD of 15 units. Though the cut-off used in assessing the test performance is identical (150 units) the degree of overlap differs. Specificity and sensitivity, of course, remain constant as these values are determined purely by the distributions of test results within the normal and abnormal patient groups.

Prevalence	Positive Predictive value	Negative predictive value
50	0.97	0.86
30	0.94	0.93
10	0.80	0.98
5	0.66	0.99
1	0.27	0.999

Figure 3.21 Effect of prevalence on test predictive value

Tests are often developed under ideal conditions with patient groups selected to show maximal contrast, sometimes for commercial reasons. Naturally this allows a test to be developed under conditions, usually of high disease prevalence, which may not be obtained in clinical practice and, therefore, published performance may not reflect that found in routine use.

Note particularly the much lower positive predictive values when the test is applied to the population with a 1% prevalence compared with that in one where the prevalence is greater than 10%. The literature is full of papers describing new tests developed in this way, tests which when applied in clinical practice fail to deliver their promise. As the diagnostics industry becomes more competitive erroneous claims of excellent performance may increase and the committed clinical scientist should treat all such claims with healthy scepticism. We discuss below criteria for the evaluation of publications concerning diagnostic tests. When reading papers relevant to the current controversies in diagnostics - e.g., third generation TSH assays, free thyroid hormones, ferritin, cardiac markers (Troponin T and Troponin I) and biochemical bone markers - it can be very instructive to check the disease prevalence in the patient groups used for evaluation and then to consider how these compare to populations that would be tested in clinical practice.

HOW ARE TEST STRATEGIES DESIGNED?

Having defined these parameters how can they be used in practice? An ideal test would have 100% sensitivity and 100% specificity. By definition this would give perfect predictive values and efficiencies. In actual practice this is very rarely achieved. If, for example, a diagnostic cut-off is set at the upper end of the 95% reference range, then by definition we will have at least 2.5% false positives and a specificity below 100%. If the diseased group overlaps with the normals, then sensitivity will be below 100%. It is possible however to adjust the performance of a test by applying different cut-offs and thus to optimally configure a test for clinical use.

MANIPULATING TEST DECISION POINTS

If we consider the case above in which we explored the effect of prevalence, what happens if we lower the upper cut-off point such that the test becomes more sensitive? We can see that the effect of this is to increase the number of false positives and thus we have to accept a trade-off of lower specificity for the test. Conversely, we could increase the cut-off to minimise the numbers of false positives, thereby increasing the specificity but at the cost of lower sensitivity.

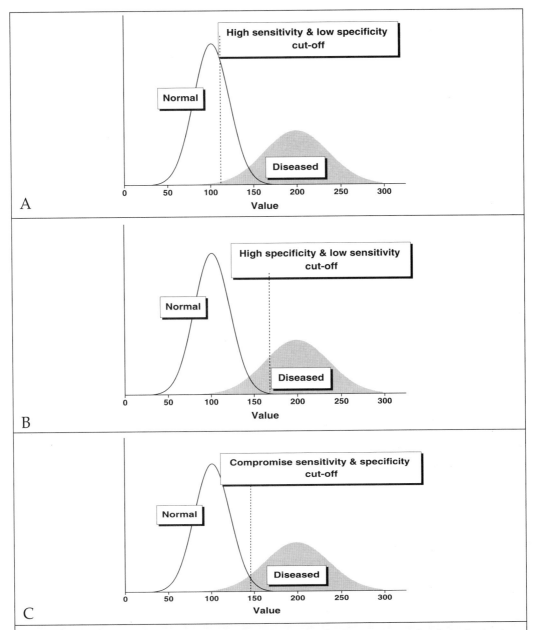

The diagnostic performance of a test can be manipulated by altering cut-off values. In the two populations shown, by shifting the cut-off to the left a high sensitivity but low specificity test may be created. Conversely, by shifting the decision point to the right a test of high specificity but low sensitivity is produced. Placing the cut-off at around the 95th centile of the normal population produces a compromise with intermediate sensitivity and specificity.

Figure 3.22 Adjusting diagnostic cut-offs

The effects of manipulating the cut-off point to change theoretical sensitivities and specificities of a test applied to a population of patients with a disease prevalence of 10% can be seen in Figure 3.23. In this case the normal population has a mean of 100 units with an SD of 25 units and the diseased population a mean of 165 units and an SD of 15 units. A high sensitivity cut off is set to 125 units and a high specificity cut-off to 170 units. One can observe the corresponding effects on the predictive values.

Cut-off (units)	False positive (%)	False negative (%)	Sensitivity (%)	Specificity (%)	Positive predictive value	Negative predictive value
125	15.9	0.4	99.6	84.1	0.411	0.999
140	5.5	4.8	95.2	94.5	0.659	0.994
150	2.3	15.9	84.1	97.7	0.804	0.982
160	0.8	36.9	63.1	99.2	0.895	0.960
170	0.3	63.1	36.9	99.7	0.941	0.934

Figure 3.23 Example of varying cut-offs to show differences in test performance

It is helpful to be able to calculate predictive values from sensitivity and specificity values to assess the usefulness of a test given different prevalences. This topic will be discussed in more detail in relation to likelihood ratios (page 110), and the relevant formulae are shown in Figure 3.24.

Positive predictive value	$\dfrac{(\text{prevalence} \times \text{sensitivity})}{(\text{prevalence} \times \text{sensitivity}) + ((1 - \text{prevalence}) \times (1 - \text{specificity}))}$
Negative predictive value	$\dfrac{((1 - \text{prevalence}) \times \text{specificity})}{((1 - \text{prevalence}) \times \text{specificity}) + (\text{prevalence} \times (1 - \text{sensitivity}))}$

Figure 3.24 Derivation of predictive values from prevalence, sensitivity and specificity

CLINICAL COST OF FALSE POSITIVES AND NEGATIVES

The exact strategy employed will depend on the desired outcome and the perceived clinical cost of false positive or false negative results. For example, if screening for a treatable disease where immediate intervention is needed and thus where missing a case would have serious irreversible consequences, then a test of high sensitivity is desirable. Tests for acute porphyria and neonatal hypothyroidism fall into this category.

Conversely, in a situation where it was important to avoid incorrect inclusion of a case because, for example, the treatment option itself carried significant risk, then a test of high specificity is more desirable. Amniocentesis coupled with cytogenetic analysis for diagnosis of Down's syndrome *in utero* is an example where this is true.

It is again important to stress that for a given test the overall performance will vary depending upon the prevalence of the abnormal state within the subject population. In Figure 3.22 we see that for a given cut-off the performance of a test alters depending on the prevalence. In Figure 3.23 we have demonstrated that by changing the cut-off the performance of a test can be altered when applied to a population with a fixed prevalence. Therefore it follows that both of these factors must be taken into account when determining how to apply a test in clinical practice. Choosing the optimum cut-off level is not always simple and a useful technique for this is the Receiver Operating Characteristic (ROC) curve, discussed in the next section.

If we now return to consider the application of reference range limits, it can be seen why these offer only a partial guide to determining the optimal use of a test. The relation of the diseased group to the normal group will significantly affect the value of a test result in identifying disease since the upper limit of normality may provide a very inappropriate cut-off in relation to diagnostic performance.

The examples of amylase and urate illustrate this well. Amylase provides a highly sensitive test if applied in an appropriate manner in the emergency situation where intra-abdominal disease is suspected. Although high values will occur in a number of other serious conditions such as mesenteric infarct, the clinical picture is likely to be such that little diagnostic confusion exists. Urate, on the other hand, demonstrates a test with little sensitivity or specificity when considered against a population reference range. Where symptoms are highly suggestive of disease however a normal or low urate value may be useful in excluding disease and allowing a more appropriate diagnostic line to be followed. These examples introduce the concept that the value of the test will depend greatly on prevailing clinical circumstances, an issue explored in more detail later.

RECEIVER OPERATING CHARACTERISTIC (ROC) CURVES
ROC curve analysis was developed as a tool to aid in the understanding of the performance of radar systems, as it allows the identification of optimal detection thresholds of operators for signals against background noise. It can be applied to clinical measurements in order to identify optimum test cut-off values, but more importantly to allow the efficacy of different tests to be compared across the full range of diagnostic decision points.

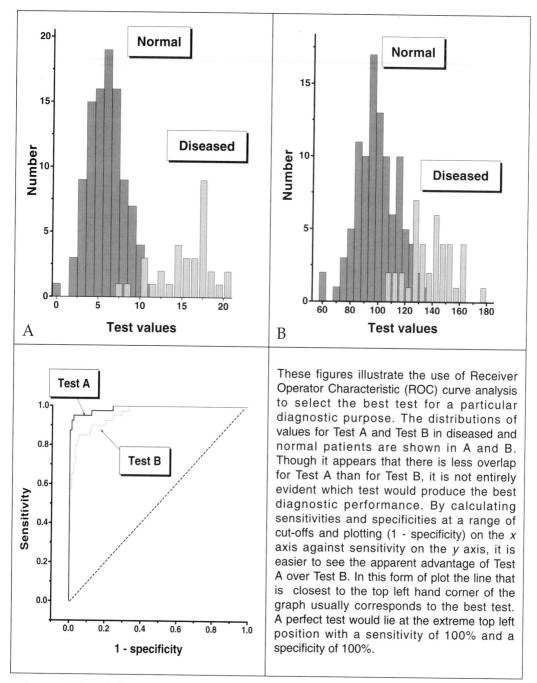

Figures 3.25   ROC curve analysis

These figures illustrate the use of Receiver Operator Characteristic (ROC) curve analysis to select the best test for a particular diagnostic purpose. The distributions of values for Test A and Test B in diseased and normal patients are shown in A and B. Though it appears that there is less overlap for Test A than for Test B, it is not entirely evident which test would produce the best diagnostic performance. By calculating sensitivities and specificities at a range of cut-offs and plotting (1 - specificity) on the x axis against sensitivity on the y axis, it is easier to see the apparent advantage of Test A over Test B. In this form of plot the line that is closest to the top left hand corner of the graph usually corresponds to the best test. A perfect test would lie at the extreme top left position with a sensitivity of 100% and a specificity of 100%.

The test is based on a graphical representation of sensitivity plotted against 1 - specificity for a range of threshold values. Tests with poor performance tend towards the 45° diagonal, whereas those with good performance curve upward and leftward. Optimum cut-off values are then evident as being the best combined value for highest sensitivity when traded against specificity, i.e. the test cut-off related to top-leftmost point on the graph. When more than one test is plotted that describing the curve furthest from the diagonal is usually the best. In making such judgements the relative cost of false positives and false negatives must be taken into account and so this rule does not apply universally as discussed in detail earlier.

The main advantage of ROC curves is the ability to display performance across the whole range of potential diagnostic cut-offs. The trade-off between sensitivity and specificity can be appreciated visually which helps when trying to decide the optimal diagnostic cut off to apply. When comparing tests it also demonstrates whether one test is better at all decision levels or whether by choosing different discriminant points the tests may be equivalent. When test performance values are reported as single estimates of sensitivity and specificity it is possible to find situations where seemingly inferior tests out-perform theoretically improved tests. This is often because of the selective nature of the reporting and we would recommend that ROC analysis always be performed and reported when describing test performance characteristics. Extensive use of ROC analysis has been made in assessing the diagnostic tests available for the investigation of pancreatitis and the recent papers by Kazmierczak and colleagues provide excellent examples.

The test may be extended by comparing derived values from the curves including the areas under the curves, although it is doubtful whether such formal calculations add much to visual inspection. If differences between curves are small, area differences are in any case likely to be of little importance, another case where statistically significant results may be found for clinically insignificant differences. Since ROC analysis is based on calculation of sensitivity and specificity, the same provisos apply. Test performance will vary in practice depending upon the prevalence of disease states in the populations under investigation and extrapolating from theoretical or laboratory test conditions to the routine world may not always be justified.

THE EFFECTS OF COMBINING TESTS

In addition to manipulating the characteristics of a single test it is possible to achieve improved diagnostic performance by combining tests into a composite test strategy. It is a commonly held belief that where clinical doubt exists conducting two diagnostic tests will yield better information than one. This is erroneous. When tests are combined their error rates are combined in addition to their true positive and true negative effects. The combined performance therefore is not additive. Great care must be taken when working with combined tests to ensure that expected outcomes are in fact achieved.

Multiple tests do have their place in clinical practice, however, and when used in well defined strategies can provide high specificities and sensitivities. It is important to understand how best to combine the tests to achieve such gains, especially as the effective use of combined tests can have economic as well as clinical advantages.

AND/OR STRATEGIES

The fundamental choice is whether to combine tests in a logical OR or in a logical AND manner. In the former case confirmation of a diagnosis is accepted when either test is positive and in the latter case when both tests are positive.

In general, just as there is a trade off between sensitivity and specificity for single tests, so too when tests are combined. The datasets in Figure 3.26 give the results separately and together for the use of two enzymes in the diagnosis of MI. The performance measures are shown for single use and for both methods of combined use.

Test	AST	CK	AST OR CK	AST AND CK
Sensitivity (%)	89.0	95.0	100.0	84.0
Specificity (%)	83.8	97.4	81.8	99.4
Positive predictive value	0.379	0.805	0.379	0.944
Negative predictive value	0.986	0.994	1.0	0.982
Efficiency (%)	84.3	97.2	83.6	97.9

Figure 3.26 Effects of *OR* and *AND* strategies on performance

Note that combining in the OR manner provides for increased sensitivity but at the expense of specificity whilst the AND combination increases specificity at the expense of sensitivity. Thus, in either case there is a cost to balance against the apparent improvement in performance although the extent of the effect will depend on the particular tests under consideration. There is no such thing as a free lunch, even in clinical decision making.

Just as cut-offs can be adjusted for single tests so they can be changed when combining tests and thus several stages of optimisation can be considered in designing the appropriate test combination.

PARALLEL AND SEQUENTIAL TEST STRATEGIES

From an operational point of view, when multiple tests are used they may be conducted in series or in parallel. The choice of which strategy to adopt is essentially an economic one as the order of testing can have significant effects on analytical costs. However, such costs have to be viewed in the context of the overall organisation of the hospital or laboratory where factors such as delayed diagnosis, repeated patient visits and prolonged hospital stays can be much more significant than marginal benefits gained through maximising internal laboratory efficiency.

Parallel use allows results to be used in both OR and AND combinations but requires that both tests be carried out on each patient sample. This may appear wasteful as a proportion of patients could have been positively diagnosed as diseased (OR combination - first test positive) or disease free (AND combination - first test negative) on the basis of a result from either test. In some cases however, as parallel testing can provide more rapid turn-round, the trade-off against extra cost may be acceptable.

Probably the major use of parallel testing is in the routine profiles used in general clinical chemistry. In the early days of automation large blanket profiles were the vogue as the trade-off of automation and output favoured running large numbers of tests at low marginal costs. With the growing sophistication of computer control of such instrumentation both at the level of the analyser and of the laboratory information system it has become more usual for patients to be tested using discreet organ-specific profiles. Reference ranges are derived statistically as 95% confidence intervals, so there is a 1 in 20 chance that we will obtain an 'abnormal' result from a normal individual. If combinations of unrelated tests are used this probability increases. For example, if a panel of 13 unrelated tests is applied to a normal person there is a 50% chance that an abnormal result will be found.

Serial use is potentially cheaper as it is possible to conduct second tests only when indicated by the initial test. For the OR combination it is necessary to run second tests only where the first is negative as patients with positive first tests are already classified as diseased. In the case of the AND combination second tests are required only for the positives since any patient with a negative test is by definition disease free. The trade-off for lower analytical costs may be longer turn-round times and effort is also necessary to select samples for retesting, though to some extent this can be automated.

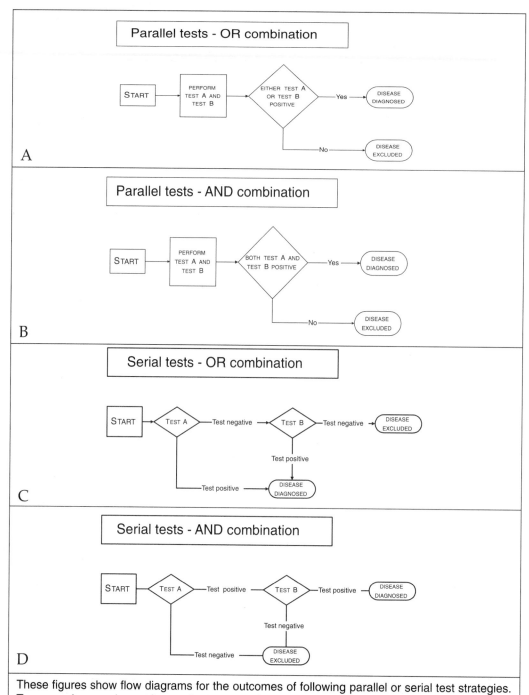

Parallel tests - OR combination

A

Parallel tests - AND combination

B

Serial tests - OR combination

C

Serial tests - AND combination

D

These figures show flow diagrams for the outcomes of following parallel or serial test strategies. Two panels are shown for each strategy showing the logic of an OR and an AND test combination.

Figures 3.27 Test strategies

COMBINATION TESTING IN NEONATAL SCREENING

The combined test approach is used to good effect in a number of practical test strategies. Neonatal screening is one area where the serial approach is adopted for economic reasons and results are combined in an AND combination to achieve high sensitivity and specificity. The challenge in the neonatal screening programmes is to identify hypothyroidism and phenylketonuria in large populations where the prevalence of disease is very low. An overall prevalence of 1 in 10000 or 0.01% has been used in the following worked example which is approximately the value for phenylketonuria (PKU).

	Total	Positive test	Negative test
Normal	99990	500	99490
Diseased	10	10	0

Sensitivity (%)	100.0
Specificity (%)	99.5
Positive predictive value	0.02
Negative predictive value	1.0
Efficiency (%)	99.5

Stage 1: First line screening for PKU using a colorimetric assay

	Total	Positive test	Negative test
Normal	500	0	500
Diseased	10	10	0

Sensitivity (%)	100.0
Specificity (%)	100.0
Positive predictive value	1.0
Negative predictive value	1.0
Efficiency (%)	100.0

Stage 2: Second line confirmation of PKU using a definitive assay

Figure 3.28   Screening test strategy for PKU

A highly sensitive test is applied at stage 1 of the investigation sequence ensuring that no cases are missed but generating a large number of false positives. The positives from test one are then screened with a highly specific test which weeds out the false positives from the true cases. Often the highly specific test will be more expensive so by taking this approach costs are reduced because the expensive test is applied to only a small percentage of the total cases.

Notice that the effect of the use of the first line test is to create a sample of higher disease prevalence (1.96%) for the application of the second test. Also it is worth remarking that under these circumstances, even though the first line test had high sensitivity and specificity, 98% of the positive tests occurred in normal patients and the positive predictive value was very low.

In this section we have explored the measures which can be used to describe diagnostic test performance and shown how they can be applied in designing and evaluating test strategies. Of particular note is the influence of disease prevalence on measures of test performance. When assessing published figures on test performance, or selecting tests for routine use, this factor must be borne in mind. The calculations involved to derive estimates of performance are mathematically trivial but can be highly revealing of flaws in the application of diagnostic tests.

HOW ARE TEST RESULTS USED IN CLINICAL PRACTICE?

Having defined the science of test optimisation, what lessons can be drawn for clinicians who are responsible for selecting tests in clinical practice?

Firstly, if the laboratory or clinical service has done its job effectively many of the factors described above will have been taken into account when developing the test repertoire and designing the format of reports, including the reference ranges, action limits, therapeutic ranges and interpretative comments. Clinicians who have any doubts about this are recommended to contact the laboratory about the service they are providing.

Given the lengths to which laboratories may have gone to optimise their tests, it follows that to get the best results, test selection at the clinical level should be equally optimised. As shown above, disease prevalence critically affects test performance and it is generally the case that optimal extra information will be provided by a test when prevalence is around 50%, rarely the case in clinical terms. For individual patients prevalence may be translated to the prior probability of disease; diagnostic tests will usually provide optimal information when the patient has a 50% chance of having the disease. Therefore, in general, tests are less likely to yield useful information when the chances of disease are small unless, that is, they have been optimised for just such a circumstance as in screening programmes. Hence chance testing - 'just in case' - is unlikely to yield worthwhile results.

A very good example of this is the routine pre-operative testing of glucose, urea and electrolytes, ECG and chest X-ray. This has become the norm in many units as clinicians have developed habits of defensive medicine. Several studies have considered this problem. In a survey of 2,785 operations the probability of identifying unsuspected and significant disease in this way was put at 0.15%. Furthermore, even in the cases where problems were identified, in only a minority did this make a difference to the clinical care provided (Kaplan *et al*, 1985). Such findings are perhaps not surprising. The prevalence of disease among the age group undergoing elective surgery is low and is better recognised on the basis of the patient's history using a few simple questions and paying attention to simple urine dipstick tests. Blanket blood testing is patently irrational and uneconomic.

At a more mundane level, if the laboratory is simply to offer age- and sex-matched reference ranges let alone provide full test interpretations, then it is important that relevant clinical demographic information is provided with the request so that these can be properly ascribed. In the absence of such information for a given patient most laboratory systems provide a default range. On occasion this may produce the effect on consecutive reports of the reference range jumping from one which is age and gender specific to a composite range. This can be potentially disconcerting unless the clinician receiving the report is aware of the way the range is assigned. Similarly, information on relevant treatments can have a profound effect on the ability of the laboratory to correctly interpret test data, erroneous conclusions being a possible result of inadequate prior information. With the increasing use of automated reflex testing and interpretation algorithms, this issue can be expected to become more prominent in future.

It is also important that samples are correctly collected and are handled and stored in an appropriate manner. Time-based reference ranges are useless for samples drawn outside the time window and where fasted ranges apply quite erroneous conclusions will be drawn from non-fasted samples. Similarly, drug samples must be taken at the appropriate time-point after a dose to prevent incorrect dose changes being instituted.

HOW CAN STATISTICS HELP INTERPRETATION OF PATIENT TEST RESULTS?

On the basis of knowledge of biological characteristics of an analyte and the performance of the assay in which it is measured, a number of useful measures to aid in the interpretation of results can be derived.

How many tests are needed to estimate the patient's true set point?

In some situations clinical treatment will be instigated when a test result crosses an action limit threshold. Since there is always a degree of uncertainty in the measure due to the combination of analytical and biological variation, it may be necessary to improve accuracy by making repeated measurements and calculating the average.

The question arises then as to how many repeated measurements are necessary to reach a confident estimate. This can be calculated from our knowledge of the analytical and intra-individual variation and the acceptable limits for the estimate.

If

n is the number of samples required,

Z is the number of standard deviates corresponding to the certainty of the estimate, 1.96 if a 95% probability is required,

CV_i + CV_a are the intra-individual and analytical coefficients of variation for the analyte in question, and

H is the percentage deviation from the homeostatic set point within which boundary we wish our estimate to lie,

then

$$n = [Z \times \sqrt{(CV_i^2 + CV_a^2)} \, / \, H]^2$$

Hence, the number will be large if we require a highly confident estimate, if the biological and/or analytical variance is high or if we wish to obtain an estimate within tight physiological bounds. This is entirely analogous to increasing our statistical confidence in a population measurement by increasing the size of the sample which is discussed in more detail in Chapters 1 and 4.

What is a clinically significant change?

Though two results from a patient may be shown to differ from a statistical point of view whether the observed difference is meaningful from a clinical point of view depends greatly on the analyte under observation and the clinical circumstances.

From the purely statistical viewpoint, the difference between two successive values has less than a 5% chance of being due to random variation if it is greater than 2.8 SDs. This figure is arrived at by what may be thought of as an inverse application of the *t*-test. A 5% probability equates to a value of *t* (two-sided) of 1.96. The formulae in Figure 3.29 show how the figure of 2.8 is derived.

$$t = \frac{\text{mean}_a - \text{mean}_b}{\sqrt{(SD_a^2 + SD_b^2)}}$$

$$1.96 = \frac{\text{mean}_a - \text{mean}_b}{\sqrt{(SD_a^2 + SD_b^2)}}$$

$$\text{mean}_a - \text{mean}_b = 1.96 \times \sqrt{(SD_a^2 + SD_b^2)}$$

Since $SD_a = SD_b$

$$\text{mean}_a - \text{mean}_b = 1.96 \times \sqrt{2(SD^2)}$$

$$= 1.96 \times \sqrt{2} \times SD$$

$$= 2.8 \times SD$$

Figure 3.29   Calculation of a statistically significant change in a test result

The SD used in making this estimate should take account of both the analytical and the intra-individual biological variation for the analyte in question. Analytical variation is sometimes much smaller than the biological variation and it is the latter figure which then has the greatest influence on the ability of sequential tests to identify a real change in test results.

Our knowledge of true values for intra-individual variation in analytes is relatively limited. It requires a far more elaborate exercise than that required to create reference ranges to collect the necessary data since multiple samples are needed from each subject. Furthermore, the fact that the degree of variation may not be constant in all circumstances makes the majority of these estimates essentially approximations. For instance, variance in an analyte may increase or decrease in the presence of a disease and such changes might occur on a disease specific basis. Indeed sometimes a change in variance is a fundamental component of the disease condition, as for example the loss of luteinising hormone (LH) pulsatility in some forms of infertility. However, having some sense of these values does help to exclude unnecessary retesting where changes are clearly small and clinically insignificant. Knowledge of the size of the effect of analytical differences alone can also help in confidently answering questions in a discussion such as 'Is the change in this value merely due to expected laboratory variation?

HOW FREQUENTLY SHOULD A TEST BE REPEATED?

Most biological substances are in a process of constant turnover where production is equal to clearance. When such processes are disturbed by illness the values of the analyte will rise or fall and on cessation of the illness will return to normal. The rate of change is commonly exponential, values halving during a fixed time period depending on the process concerned. For example following resection of the prostate for carcinoma the prostate specific antigen (PSA) value falls with a half life of about 2-3 days. Whether such a change will be recognisable depends upon the degree of variation of the analyte, the starting value and the period between tests. Repeated testing at frequent intervals at low baseline values when changes are small is unlikely to yield meaningful results and should be avoided. No hard rules exist to determine the frequency with which to conduct tests partly because our knowledge of the time course of change in biological systems is relatively weak. However, this is no excuse for the over-frequent use of tests which is so often seen in clinical practice. For example, the daily repetition of thyroid function or liver function tests which is increasing because of the easy availability of automated assays provides little or no diagnostic information since the time course of change for these systems may be measured in days or weeks.

CLINICAL EXAMPLES OF USE OF TIME-BASED INTERPRETATION

There are numerous occasions where analysis over time may provide more valuable information than single test results. Two further examples will be cited which not only take account of time-based changes but also illustrate the value of using the patient as his or her own reference point.

Plasma Creatinine - Though a population-based reference range can be determined for this variable, in practice we are often more interested in change within the individual. For an individual patient in a steady state there is little day-to-day variation in fasting plasma creatinine. Therefore small changes over time can be of significance. This is especially important when one considers the relationship between creatinine and glomerular filtration rate (GFR) which is distinctly non-linear. In Figure 3.30 we have shown two patients with similar progressive changes in creatinine. Because of the relationship of creatinine to GFR both show large falls in GFR with small increases in creatinine over the range of GFR of 40 - 140 mL/min. Patient A, who was the smaller of the two, started at a low value of creatinine and thus did not break through the upper limit of the population reference range until the GFR had fallen to 50 mL/min whereas Patient B, whose starting point was higher, presented with an abnormal result when the GFR fell to 80 mL/min.

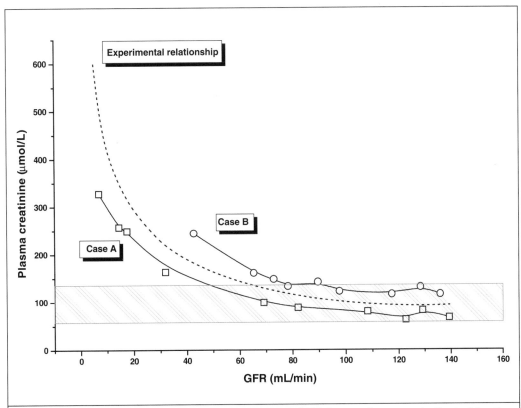

The relationship between plasma creatinine and GFR is non-linear as indicated by the experimental relationship showing the theoretical curve which would be obtained if the GFR were progressively reduced in a normal individual. Cases A and B show the results in two individuals whose GFR falls at the same absolute rate over a period of time. Note that, because Case B starts at a higher base line of creatinine, the patient breaks through the normal upper limit of the reference range at a GFR of 80 mL/minute. As Case A starts with a lower creatinine value they break through the upper reference range at a level much lower of GFR (50 mL/minute). For a given plasma creatinine there may be a wide range of GFR. This shows that a within-patient change in creatinine levels, even within the reference range, may provide more significant diagnostic information of renal deterioration than the absolute value of a single measurement.

Figure 3.30 Plasma creatinine and GFR

One way around the problem is to generate individualised reference ranges taking into account factors such as age, gender and weight but this requires close co-ordination between clinical and laboratory activities, beyond that generally practised to date. A softer approach is to issue cumulative results with comments on the significance of change hoping that clinicians are aware of the underlying physiological problem and therefore are alert to the possibility of missing the early diagnosis of progressive renal damage.

As an aside, although fasting plasma creatinine is relatively stable, non-fasting plasma and urine creatinines are sufficiently affected by other factors including diet to make them unsuitable for the accurate measurement of creatinine clearance as a substitute for GFR. Many clinicians are under the misapprehension that creatinine clearance provides a more accurate estimate of renal function than fasting plasma creatinine alone. The errors inherent in the measurement of creatinine clearance are larger than for creatinine alone and there is good evidence that better diagnostic information is provided by proper appreciation of the interpretation of the simple blood test, as indicated above, than from the application of the pseudoscience of creatinine clearance.

Serum cardiac markers in myocardial infarction (CK, CK-MB, Troponin) - The diagnosis of myocardial infarction is classically based on a pattern of change of CK over time with a rise and fall being observed over 2-3 days. An alternative approach is to consider the rate of change as the diagnostic parameter, which it is claimed, allows an increase in both the precision of the diagnostic test and the speed of availability of the diagnostic result. Since a rate is used the value is actually baseline independent and thus, effectively, patients are used as their own control level. Further, as the time zero is set as the time of the first test the result is independent of the time after the onset of symptoms. This allows the diagnostic window to be extended to an earlier point in the clinical episode than is true with conventional testing where tests in the first 6 hours are generally uninformative as, in most infarct patients, cardiac marker values will be in the reference range even though they may be rising. With modern tests the minimum window for diagnosis falls to 4 hours, still arguably outside the diagnostic time-frame required for the clinical decision as to whether to commence thrombolysis, but rapid enough to reduce the number of patients receiving an extended and unnecessary course of a potentially harmful therapy. For a fuller discussion of these concepts see Scott *et al* and Johnston *et al* (See Further reading).

Analyte	Between day analytical CV (%)	Between day biological CV (%)	Combined CV (%)	Between day real change at $P<0.05$ (%)	Example of changes	Typical desirable clinical precision	Number of samples for true baseline
Sodium	1.0	0.7	1.2	3.4	5 mmol/L @ 140 mmol/L	2 mmol/L (1.4%)	4
Potassium	1.8	5.1	5.4	15	0.6 mmol/L @ 4.0 mmol/L	0.2 mmol/L (5%)	5
Urea	6.6	13.6	15.1	42	2.1 mmol/L @ 5.0 mmol/L	0.2 mmol/L (4%)	55
Creatinine	8.5	4.6	9.7	27	23 μmol/L @ 85 μmol/L	5 μmol/L (6%)	10
Calcium	1.0	1.7	2.0	5.5	0.13 mmol/L @ 2.4 mmol/L	0.05 mmol/L (2%)	4
Phosphate	4.0	7.8	8.8	24.5	0.25 mmol/L @ 1.0 mmol/L	0.1 mmol/L (10%)	3
Albumin	1.5	3.1	3.4	9.6	4 g/L @ 40 g/L	1 g/L (2.5%)	7
Cholesterol	2.3	5.5	6.0	16.6	1.0 mmol/L @ 7.0 mmol/L	0.2 mmol/L (3%)	15

Figure 3.31 Typical average day-to-day variability for some analytes, with the calculated between-day real change and numbers of samples needed to estimate a true baseline at typical desirable levels of clinical precision

HOW CAN KNOWLEDGE OF TEST RESULTS PROVIDE CLINICALLY USEFUL INFORMATION?

USING INFORMATION ABOUT PREVALENCE

We have seen how positive and negative predictive values can be calculated for a given test to provide an indication of the probability that a patient with a given test result will or will not have the disease in question. The underlying assumption is that the patient's baseline risk was the same as that in the population from which the reference range was drawn. In practice this is rarely true and allowance must be made for the individuals degree of initial risk. This is known as the *pre-test odds*. By combining it with the results of a test a modified risk estimate, the *post-test odds* that the patient actually has the disease in question, can be calculated.

Take, for example, the case when a patient is selected from a group where 25% are at risk of having a disease, that is the prevalence is 25%. The *pre-test odds* of an individual patient having the disease is the ratio of the chance that the patient has the disease to the chance that the patient does not have the disease. In the absence of data about an individual's risk factors the former is approximately equal to prevalence and by definition the latter must be (1 - prevalence). Thus the *pre-test odds* is prevalence / (1 - prevalence) which in this case is 0.33 or 3 to 1 against the disease being present.

To calculate the post-test odds this value is modified using the *likelihood ratio*. This is defined as the ratio between the probability of finding a positive test in the presence of a disease to the probability of a positive test in the absence of the disease.

Presented graphically, this is the ratio of the probabilities of positivity in diseased and normal patients represented by the heights of the corresponding probability density curves at the value of the test measured. Where the curves can be modelled to fit Normal distributions this can be calculated mathematically and readers are referred to Sackett *et al* for more detailed information (See Further Reading).

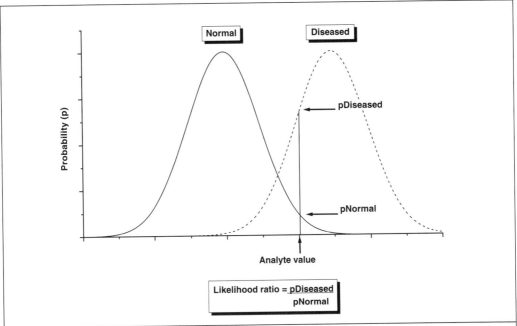

The likelihood ratio is derived from knowledge of the distribution of test results in the normal and diseased population. The probability of disease in any particular individual corresponds to the height of the diseased population distribution at the patient's analyte value and the probability that individual is normal corresponds to the height of the normal population distribution at the same analyte value. In this example the patient has a lower probability of normality than of disease. The ratio of the two probabilities is the likelihood ratio. It can be seen that for very low analyte values this likelihood ratio would be very small as the probability of disease tends to zero. As the analyte value increases the likelihood ratio increases as the probability of normality is much diminished. By combining the likelihood ratio with the known prior probability of disease, the risk for an individual patient can be assessed. In some circumstances likelihood ratios can be derived for a number of analytes simultaneously and the results combined. A good example of this is the Triple Test used for Down's Syndrome Screening.

Figure 3.32 The likelihood ratio

A calculation which is often used to devise the approximate likelihood ratio for a test is to divide the true positive rate (sensitivity) of the test by the false positive rate (1 - specificity). Technically this is known as the *likelihood ratio positive* to distinguish it from directly derived individual values.

$$\text{Likelihood ratio positive} = \frac{\% \text{ Positive tests in diseased patients}}{\% \text{ Positive tests in healthy patients}} = \frac{\% \text{ Sensitivity}}{100 - \% \text{ Specificity}}$$

Figure 3.33 Likelihood ratio positive

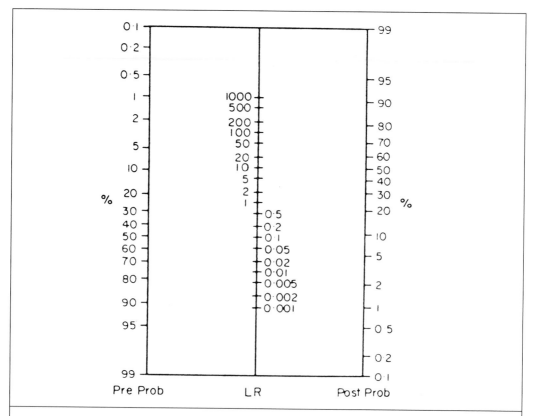

This nomogram is a useful way of combining likelihood ratios with prior probabilities to obtain the likelihood of disease in an individual patient. A line is drawn from the prior (pre-test) probability of disease on the left scale through the likelihood ratio in the centre scale to obtain the post-test probability from the right-hand scale. It should be clear from this graph that unless likelihood ratios are either large (>10) or small (<0.1) they make little impression upon the probability of disease in individual patients. In other words tests with intermediate likelihood ratios are unlikely to provide useful diagnostic information.

From: Sackett D L, Haynes R B, Guyatt G H, Tugwell P. *Clinical Epidemiology: a Basic Science for Clinical Medicine*, 2nd edn. Boston: Little, Brown and Company, 1991

Figure 3.34 Using likelihood ratios to aid diagnosis

It should be pointed out that the likelihood ratio positive can give erroneous results in some circumstances as it provides an average picture and does not take into account how far a result lies from the decision point. Where likelihood ratios are calculated mathematically from derived curves, for example in calculating antenatal risks for Down's Syndrome in triple-test screening programmes, such evidence is included in the calculation of a highly individualised test result.

To return to our example of a patient with pre-test odds of 0.33. If the sensitivity of the test was 0.85 (85%) and the specificity 0.70 (70%), then the likelihood ratio positive is 2.83 and the *post-test odds* of the patient having the disease given a positive test would shorten to 0.93 or nearly evens (0.33 x 0.85 / (1 - 0.7)). On the other hand, if the prevalence were 10% the patient would have an initial risk of only 0.11 and the *post-test odds* would be 0.31, that is a 1 to 3 chance of disease. If the prevalence were as low as 1% then the final risk turns out to be only 0.0283 or a 1 to 35 chance of disease, only a little better than the initial risk. Put another way, where diseases are uncommon it is still more likely that a patient with a positive test will be normal than abnormal. This is another way of demonstrating that the usefulness of test may be determined almost entirely by the disease prevalence which equates to the pre-test odds.

From the apparent circularity of these arguments it may be tempting to conclude that the application of the concepts of positive and negative predictive values and likelihood ratios are unhelpful. This would be a false conclusion. The effects demonstrated are important in understanding test efficacy and its appropriate application. Turning the argument on its head, for a test to be useful in the diagnosis of a low prevalence condition as usually obtained in a screening programme, very high sensitivities and specificities are required to produce meaningful data.

Sensitivity %	Specificity %	Likelihood ratio positive given a positive test
70	70	2.3
80	80	4
90	90	9
99	90	9.9
99.9	90	9.99
90	95	18
99	95	19.8
99.9	95	19.98
90	99	90
99	99	99
99.9	99	99.9

Figure 3.35 Likelihood ratio positive for a series of sensitivities and specificities

It should be clear from Figure 3.35 that the specificity of the test is the most important determinant of the likelihood ratio positive for a given range of test sensitivities. Since the likelihood ratio is used as a multiplier in the calculation of post-test odds, it can be seen that it will have a significant effect in changing initial low pre-test odds only at higher values of sensitivity and specificity. The first two rows in the Figure provide likelihood ratios positive at levels of test sensitivity and specificity which are commonly found in published papers. It is not hard to see why many claims of test efficacy made in the literature do not translate into clinical performance.

Likelihood ratios come into their own in cases where the combination of information from several tests is required. Consider the case of a sequential test strategy where a disease prevalence is 10%. A patient thus has a *pre-test odds* of 1 to 9 or 0.11. A positive first test where the sensitivity is 99.9% and specificity 98% increases the odds of disease to 5.495 (i.e. 0.11 x 0.999 / (1 - 0.98)) or 5.5 to 1 that the disease is present. Applying a second test of sensitivity 99% but specificity 99.9% which proves positive increases the odds that the patient has the disease to 5440 to 1 (i.e. 5.495 x 0.99 / (1 - 0.999)). This is akin to the analysis made above to sequential test strategies used in screening programmes.

BAYES' THEOREM

The above approach is an example of the use of Bayes' theorem which allows independent probabilities to be associated with a *prior probability* to give a combined risk, equivalent to the *pre-test* and *post-test odds* discussed above. In the case of diseases and tests this amounts to taking the prior risk (the *prior odds*), often based on knowledge of prevalence, and combining it with the extra information provided by a test result to give an individualised risk (often called the *posterior odds*) for a patient.

Posterior odds = Prior odds x Likelihood ratio

The application of Bayes' theorem depends on many assumptions such as the results of the tests being statistically independent and in practice the mathematics can become quite tortuous. However the concept has been extensively used in clinical decision support systems with some major successes such as the acute abdominal pain diagnostic system of the late Professor de Dombal.

Probably the most widely used laboratory application of these techniques is the Triple Test used for the screening for Down's syndrome *in utero*. The prior risk in this case is taken as the age-related risk of a mother carrying a Down's foetus and this is modified by a likelihood ratio calculated from the known values of biochemical tests in affected and unaffected pregnancies. In practice the calculation is complex as several test results are combined and allowance has to be made for the interactions which exist between them. For a clear explanation of the mathematics involved see Reynolds *et al*.

A convenient way of using likelihood ratio data is to use a nomogram first published in the New England Journal of Medicine in 1975 and later modified as in Fig 3.34. The patient's initial risk is plotted on the left axis, the likelihood ratio in the centre axis and the final risk is obtained by extrapolating to the right hand axis. It can be seen that likelihood ratios of 10 or above produce meaningful and useful modifications of initial risk. If it is known that a test being conducted to aid diagnosis will not provide a likelihood ratio of this magnitude, then it is unlikely to provide extra useful information.

This nomogram can be used when combining the information from tests by treating the post-test risks from one test as the pre-test risk for the next. Although strictly speaking likelihood ratios used in combination should be statistically independent, in practice the degree of distortion is not great even when they are not. However, caution is urged especially when using the potential error inherent in the likelihood ratio positive.

The application of likelihood ratios positive for a particular test is very laboratory-dependent. Their use depends to a great extent on the prevalence of diseases under investigation in the local population and on the reference ranges and analytical characteristics of the laboratory's methods. A useful list of typical likelihood ratios for use in these types of calculation can be found in Panzer. It should be recognised, however, that the best approach is to ensure close liaison between the laboratory and its clinicians so that knowledge of local circumstances can be fully incorporated into the process of diagnostic decision making.

USING THE RESULTS OF CLINICAL TRIALS
Several methods may be used to summarise the outcomes of randomised clinical trials where interventions have been tested against placebo. Most clinical trials are reported in relation to the improvement in patient well being due to the treatment intervention. The most usual statistical measure used is the *relative risk reduction* due to the treatment compared with placebo control, sometimes expressed as an *odds ratio*.

The absolute risk reduction is the proportion of patients suffering the outcome of interest in the control group (x) minus the proportion of patients suffering the same outcome in the treatment group (y). The outcome in the control group (x) is effectively the background risk.

The relative risk is the ratio of these proportions (y/x).

The relative risk reduction is the relative difference in outcome expressed in percentage terms, $((x - y) / x) \times 100$.

An odds ratio is the ratio of the odds that the outcome of interest will occur in patients in as compared to the treatment control groups. Mathematically this is defined as $(y / (1y)) / (x / (1 - x))$. Where the outcomes of interest occur in less than 10% of the patients in both groups, the odds ratio approximates to the relative risk and may be used as such in further calculations.

The term risk is used because these measures were first developed in epidemiological studies where the intervention being studied was usually a deleterious environmental factor. On occasion we may be interested in an increase in events in the intervention group as a result of treatment, for example, increased numbers of patients giving up smoking as a result of using nicotine patches. A relative risk greater than 1.0 then indicates treatment benefit.

As an example, if a group of asthmatics treated with steroid inhalers in addition to bronchodilators were compared with a group taking only the latter, we could estimate the number of patients in whom asthma attacks had been prevented.

	Bronchodilators	**Bronchodilators + steroids**
Attacks present	60	61
Attacks absent	10	39
No of patients	70	100
Attack risk	x = 60/70 = 0.86	y = 61/100 = 0.61

Table 3.36 Asthma attack risk with two treatments

The absolute risk reduction for these patients is the difference between the proportions suffering asthma attacks in the two groups, in this case 0.25 (i.e. 0.86 - 0.61).

The relative risk is the ratio of the proportion of affected individuals in the intervention group to the proportion of affected individuals in the control group, in this case 0.71 (i.e. 0.61 / 0.86) pointing to an improvement due to the steroids.

The relative risk reduction is derived from these figures by expressing the difference in risk as a proportion of the risk in the control group ((0.86 - 0.61) / 0.86) x 100. In this case the *relative risk reduction* is 29.1%.

THE NUMBER NEEDED TO TREAT

Though meaningful to statisticians and epidemiologists, these risk values are sometimes difficult to interpret because unfortunately the measures of *relative risk reduction* do not include information on the background rate of events in the patients groups. Thus it may be difficult to appreciate the true worth of an intervention in relation to routine clinical practice. What does a *relative risk reduction* of 29.1% actually mean for individual patients? Are they 29.1% less likely to get an attack? Are 29.1% more of the total number of patients going to be attack free with the intervention than without it? An alternative measure which can be derived from these values is the Number Needed to Treat (NNT) which helps to put this data into a working clinical context. It has been promoted as being much easier for non-specialists to understand.

NNT is defined as the number of patients who would need to be treated by a particular intervention to see benefit in at least one of them *because of that intervention.* Note that because placebo effects may be large and variable, it is important to differentiate the "treatment-specific" NNT from the overall proportion that might improve. In mathematical terms the number needed to treat is the reciprocal of the *absolute risk reduction*. From the calculations for asthmatics above this works out at 4.0 (i.e. 1.0 / 0.25). This means that for every 4 asthmatics treated with steroids in addition to broncho-dilators we would expect to see one more in whom attacks would be prevented.

This measure is useful in summarising the information from clinical trials as it presents the information in a manner which is more easily understood in terms of patient benefit. The term takes account of the background risk and thus is useful in comparing results across a range of disease prevalences.

The calculation of NNT from the numbers who have shown improvement in a control and an active treatment group is summarised in Figure 3.37. Note that because the concept being considered is a reduction of risk it is possible to get negative values when the risk is increased (or where data has been inadvertently transposed).

THE EFFECT OF BASELINE RISK

Just as test efficacies vary with the prevalence of illness in the subject population so the benefits of interventions are affected by the baseline risk of patients. The NNT measure is

	Control group (c)	Active group (a)
Number improved (I)	Ic	Ia
Total number of patients (N)	Nc	Na
Proportion improved in control group (x)	Ic / Nc	
Proportion improved in active group (y)	Ia / Na	
Relative Risk (RR)	x / y	
Relative Risk Reduction (RRR)	((x - y) / x) x 100	
Absolute Risk Reduction (ARR)	x - y	
Number Needed to Treat (NNT)	1 / ARR = 1 / (x - y)	

useful for revealing and controlling for these effects.

Figure 3.37 Calculation of the Number Needed to Treat

For example, consider two situations where the same relative risk reduction has been observed but where the initial risks are different. Suppose a treatment causes a reduction in the rate of MI in a group of patients from 0.20 in the control group to 0.12 in the intervention group. The relative risk reduction is 40%. The absolute risk reduction is 0.08. Thus, in order to prevent the MI in one additional patient, a total of 13 would have to be treated.

By contrast, consider another situation where the baseline risk is lower but where the same relative risk reduction can be achieved by the same treatment. In this case the baseline risk of MI is 0.015 in controls and a rate of MI of 0.009 is observed in the treated group. The same relative risk reduction of 40% ((1.5 - 0.9) x 100) / 1.5) is present between the treated and control patients. However, in this case there is a much lower absolute risk reduction, 0.006, and a correspondingly greater NNT. In fact the NNT is more than 10 times greater and 150 patients would require treatment in order to prevent one adverse event.

The major difference between the groups is the much lower prevalence of the disease state in the second group, the first group being hypertensive smokers and the second group normotensive non-smokers. Therefore, as would be expected intuitively, in order to see a reduction of events of similar magnitude more patients need to be treated. To see a significant change in an event which happens infrequently requires highly effective interventions. Also, if the intervention itself carries risk then clearly justification of its use is harder for the latter low prevalence group than the former high prevalence group.

COMPARING AND COMBINING RISK ASSESSMENTS

The NNT is particularly useful when attempting to balance the risks of intervention of a particular treatment against the perceived benefit because it shows the change in risk in terms of numbers of patients treated. The NNT can be directly compared with the known risks of a treatment. For example, if 1 in 100 patients suffer an adverse effect from a drug, its use would be justified only if the NNT for benefit were at a substantially lower value.

The NNT is also helpful when trying to make comparisons between different interventions. It has been used, for example, in comparisons of the efficacy of different anti-emetic preparations or different pain relieving agents. By calculating the NNT for each intervention it is possible to produce a rank ordering of the effectiveness of the various agents under comparison, and therefore to assess whether one treatment is better than another.

By rigorously applying this method it is therefore possible to assess whether exaggerated claims in terms of percentage improvement in performance will actually be significant in practice. Furthermore, it provides a scale of measurement against which other risks, such as those of adverse events, can be weighed. In this way relatively straightforward cost-benefit comparisons become feasible. For further discussion see copies of *Bandolier*, available from Editorial Office, Pain Relief Unit, The Churchill, Oxford OX3 7LF, UK or on the World Wide Web (http://www.jr2.ox.ac.uk/Bandolier). The website of the Centre for Evidence Based Medicine, Oxford, UK (http://cebm.jr2.ox.ac.uk/docs/newindex.html) also carries a great deal of useful, related information.

SUMMARY

This section has covered the theoretical basis of test design and use. We have steered a course from a working scientific definition of 'normality' through to a discussion of the descriptive parameters of clinical tests to an analysis of how tests and their results may be optimised for clinical use. In the final analysis fine judgement is needed to selecting the correct approach for a particular application. Knowing how to trade off different aspects of performance one against another to arrive at the best compromise takes experience and skill. Of fundamental importance is the understanding that tests form only one component of the clinical process. If they are to be designed, developed, tested and used successfully then the clinician and laboratory specialist alike must appreciate their strengths and weaknesses and must always consider the context in which they are used before reaching conclusions about the reliability of the information they generate.

If there is a single recurrent theme it is that the underlying prevalence of disease critically determines the value of a test and the approach that must be taken during test development. Just as with the classical statistical methods described in Chapters 1 and 2, the conceptual challenge in diagnostic testing is to confidently separate signal from noise. Where signal levels are low, precise and accurate tests are needed to give confident answers. Low prevalence equates to low signal and by analogy creates the need to apply powerful tests to generate robust clinical information.

FURTHER READING

Balla J, Iansek R, Elstein A. Bayesian diagnosis in presence of pre-existing disease. *Lancet* 1985; I: 326-30

Barth J H, Fiddy J B, Payne R B. Adjustment of serum total calcium for albumin concentration: effects of non-linearity and of regression differences between laboratories. *Ann Clin Biochem* 1996; **33**: 55-58

Bucher H C, Weinbacher M, Gyr K. Influence of method of reporting study results on decision of physicians to prescribe drugs to lower cholesterol concentration. *Br Med J* 1994; **309**: 761-4

Cook R J, Sackett D L. The number needed to treat: a clinically useful measure of treatment effect. *Br Med J* 1995; 310: 452-4 (see also erratum in *Br Med J* 1995; 310: 1056) de Dombal F T. Computer-aided diagnosis and decision-making in the acute abdomen. *J R Coll Physicians Lond* 1975; **9:** 211-8

Expert Panel on Theory of Reference Values (EPTRV), International Federation of Clinical Chemistry, Scientific Committee, Clinical Section. The theory of reference values. Part 5. Statistical treatment of collected reference values. Determination of reference limits. *Clin Chim Acta* 1984; **137:** 97F-114F

Fagan T J. Nomogram for Bayes' theorem (letter). *N Engl J Med* 1975; **293:** 257

Harris E K, Boyd, J C. *Statistical Bases of Reference Values in Laboratory Medicine.* New York: Marcel Dekker Inc, 1995

Galen R S, Gambino S R. *Beyond Normality: The Predictive Value and Efficiency of Medical Diagnoses.* New York: John Wiley and Sons, 1995

Garcia-Romero H, Garcia-Barrios C, Ramos-Gutierrez F. Effects of uncertain results on sensitivity and specificity of diagnostic tests. *Lancet* 1996; **348:** 1745-6.

Hallworth M, Capps N. *Therapeutic Drug Monitoring and Clinical Biochemistry.* London: ACB Venture Publications, 1993

Henderson A R. Assessing test accuracy and its clinical consequences: a primer for receiver operating characteristic curve analysis. *Ann Clin Biochem* 1993; **30:** 521-39

Johnston J D, Collinson P O, Rosalki S B. MIDAS: myocardial infarct diagnosis by assessment of slope. *Ann Clin Biochem* 1993; **30:** 407-9

Kazmierczak S C, Catrou P G, Van Lente F. Enzymatic markers of gallstone-induced pancreatitis identified by ROC curve analysis, discriminant analysis, logistic regression, likelihood ratios, and information theory. *Clin Chem* 1995; **41:** 523-31

Kazmierczak S C, Catrou P G, Van Lente F. Diagnostic accuracy of pancreatic enzymes evaluated by use of multivariate data analysis. *Clin Chem* 1993; **39:** 1960-5

Kaplan E B, Sheiner L B, Boeckmann A J, *et al.* The usefulness of preoperative laboratory screening. *JAMA* 1985; **253:** 3576-81

Little A J, Williams R B, Parker S D, Payne RB. The derivation of biochemical normal ranges from a hospital outpatient population. *Clin Chim Acta* 1974; **57:** 91-95

Panzer R J, Black E R, Griner P F. *Diagnostic Strategies for Common Medical Problems.* Philadelphia, American College of Physicians, 1991

Payne R B, Jones D P, Walker A P, Evans R T. Clustering of serum calcium and magnesium concentrations in siblings. *Clin Chem* 1986; **32:** 349-50

Reynolds T M, Penney M D. The mathematical basis of multivariate risk screening: with special reference to screening for Down's syndrome associated pregnancy. *Ann Clin Biochem* 1990; **27:** 452-8 (see also *Br Med J* 1995; **310:** 452)

Riegelman R, Schroth W S. Adjusting the number needed to treat: incorporating adjustments for the utility and timing of benefits and harms. *Med Decis Making* 1993; **13**: 247-52

Sackett D L, Haynes R B, Guyatt G H, Tugwell P. *Clinical Epidemiology: a Basic Science for Clinical Medicine*, 2nd edn. Boston: Little, Brown and Company, 1991

Scott B B, Simmons A V, Newton K E, Payne R B. Interpretation of serum creatine kinase in suspected myocardial infarction. *Br Med J* 1974; **4**: 691-3

UK Collaborative Study. Maternal serum alpha-fetoprotein measurement in the antenatal screening for anencephaly and spina bifida in early pregnancy. *Lancet* 1997; **i**: 1323-32

White R H, Mungall D. Outpatient management of warfarin therapy: comparison of computer- predicted dosage adjustment to skilled professional care. *Ther Drug Monit* 1991; **13**: 46-50

AUSTIN BRADFORD HILL

Born 8 July 1897. Died 18 April 1991.

As a schoolboy 'Tony' Bradford Hill had hoped to study medicine. However, during service in the first world war he developed pulmonary tuberculosis and at the age of 19 was invalided home to die. Fortunately he improved after an artificial pneumothorax and was able to study for an external BSc in economics while convalescing. He subsequently undertook epidemiological research with an MRC grant, and attended the BSc course in statistics in Karl Pearson's department at University College, London. In 1923 he joined the staff of the MRC and was a member of its Industrial Health Research Board. In 1933 he was appointed Reader in the Department of Medical Statistics in the London School of Hygiene. In 1945 he succeeded to the Chair and also became Honorary Director of the MRC Statistical Research Unit, posts which he held until his retirement in 1961. In that year he received a knighthood.

His close colleague, Prof. Sir Richard Doll, believed that Bradford Hill had a greater influence than many winners of the Nobel prize for medicine because of the impact his teachings had on the development of medical science. His lectures on statistics at the London School of Hygiene and at the Postgraduate Medical School were published as a series of 17 articles in the *Lancet* in 1937 and then reprinted as a book, *Principles of Medical Statistics*. This had an enormous effect both on the design of medical investigations and on the interpretation of results. The 12th edition, with one of his sons as co-author, was published in the year of his death, 1991.

His investigations with Richard Doll of the relationship between smoking and lung cancer provided outstanding models for both retrospective case control studies and prospective cohort studies. In 1947 he helped to design the MRC investigation of the efficacy of streptomycin in the treatment of tuberculosis as the first double blind randomised controlled trial. Randomisation, which had been used by Ronald Fisher in agricultural research, thereafter became obligatory in medical research.

Bradford Hill's teachings were widely and rapidly accepted, not only because of their intrinsic worth but also because of his skills as a communicator. His lectures were models of clarity and usually not without humour. He was a quiet, unassuming person with a razor sharp intelligence. He did have one blind spot: it is said that he retired a little early to avoid the computer.

Chapter 4

Medical Research: Study design, analysis and reporting

INTRODUCTION

"I have yet to see any problem, however complicated which when you looked at it in the right way did not become still more complicated."

Poul Anderson

Anyone pursuing a career in the higher specialist grades of clinical medicine will be expected to have undertaken practical research work. A period of research activity has also been a major element of clinical scientific training for clinical scientists and pathologists. The assumption is that, by experiencing research at first hand, individuals will acquire the skills needed to evaluate experimental data and therefore be better able to judge the worth of new ideas and approaches. The current trend towards the practice of 'evidence-based medicine' will demand that all clinicians and clinical scientists have a thorough grounding in the principles of good experimental design and an ability to interpret data originating in clinical studies.

Hospital laboratories play an important role in clinical research and are often the first port of call for clinicians who are setting up studies. Laboratory medical staff and scientists are expected to provide research support to colleagues. They are often amongst the most highly trained scientific personnel in a hospital and can act as a valuable source of advice on study design and clinical data analysis. It is therefore doubly important for such staff to have a thorough grounding in research techniques.

Formal training in research methodology has not been prominent in undergraduate or post-graduate medical training and most people have been expected to pick up research experience 'on the side'. Times are changing however. Many PhD programmes now include a taught element providing such training and courses in research methodology are more commonly available.

Attendance on such a course is strongly recommended for the novice researcher who should be aiming to acquire the following essential skills:

- The ability to read research papers critically.
- The ability to recognise and devise significant questions.
- Knowledge of the ethical issues involved in experimentation.
- The ability to apply for funding.
- Knowledge of when and how to apply statistical tests.
- The ability to present data as tables and graphs.
- The ability to present research findings verbally and in writing.

Chapter 4 will provide an introduction to the principles of study design and execution and hopefully will act as a primer for more detailed study of this important aspect of scientific activity.

WHAT ARE THE CLASSIC TYPES OF STUDY DESIGN?

There are a multitude of different study designs; indeed, in most cases studies need to be custom-designed for each particular scientific question. For some researchers the development of study designs has become a science in its own right. The recent expansion of the use of meta-analysis has lead to heated controversies about the appropriate ways in which to combine data and also has lead to more rigorous appraisal of the designs of primary studies. In broad terms there are two categories of studies.

Observational studies answer questions such as:

What is the value of a test result in a population of patients?

Do the results of a test in a study population differ from those in a control group?

What proportion of patients over 65 have hypercalcaemia?

Interventional studies are designed to answer questions such as:

Does treatment a change outcome b?

Is treatment x more effective than treatment y?

Does treatment with anti-thrombotic agents reduce the incidence of myocardial infarction?

Does the availability of near-patient testing improve the treatment of diabetics?

Observational studies estimate values which exist in populations of subjects or in collections of materials such as laboratory specimens. They are used to describe the current state of affairs and may allow conclusions to be drawn as to the importance of events or the conditions which affect the population or materials. They may also be able to identify associations between events and draw hypotheses about causative links where y may follow from x. Proof of causation can only be obtained through intervention studies however, as it is rare for an experiment of nature to provide ideal conditions for such analysis.

In *intervention* studies the effects of controlled manipulations are observed from measurements made before and after the event, so conclusions may be drawn about causality or effectiveness. Indeed, experimental conditions may be manipulated specifically to aid such analysis. Intervention studies tend to be more elaborate in design as, in order to improve their power, it is necessary to control as many potentially confounding factors as possible. In effect this improves the accuracy of the measurements made (the signal) by reducing random errors (the noise).

In recent years an additional distinction has been drawn between intervention studies which are *evaluative* and those which are *pragmatic*. In the former the experimental aim is to increase understanding of the problem, for example whether prophylactic treatment with antibiotics can influence peri-operative infections. In the latter the aim is to decide the best approach to adopt to solve a particular medical problem, for example to decide which antibiotic to use to prevent peri-operative infection. The difference may appear subtle but with the growth of interest in evidence-based medicine the adoption of the pragmatic approach will become more common. This distinction is discussed in more detail below.

Study Type	Outcome
Observation	Estimation and description Assessment of group differences Identification of association
Intervention: evaluative	Study of treatments / actions Proof of causation
Intervention: pragmatic	Assessment of treatments / actions Proof of effectiveness

Figure 4.1 Study types and outcomes

Study type	Description	Definition
Observation	Population census analysis	Studies where data from routinely collected sources, e.g. hospital discharge returns, are analysed retrospectively.
Observation	Cohort studies	Studies in which groups of patients are identified and followed up over time. The patient selection occurs at the point of entry and is usually based upon demographic criteria or exposure to an environmental or medical event.
Observation	Case control studies	Studies in which experimental cases are compared with control cases which are matched for factors other than that under examination, e.g. age and sex matched controls for patients presenting with myocardial infarction. The patient selection is usually based upon the presence of an outcome or medical endpoint such as the presence of a disease or morbid state. Controls are then retrospectively matched.
Observation	Surveys	Studies in which data are collected from populations often by analysis of existing databases or by questionnaire. This is the simplest form of observational study and might be used to identify, for example, the prevalence or incidence of a particular disease within a defined population.
Observation	Cross sectional study	Short term studies where data is collected over a narrow time slice. This may be in the form of a retrospective observational study.
Observation	Method comparisons	Studies where two or more methods of measurement of the same variable measured in the same materials or on the same subjects are compared.

Figure 4.2 Examples of study types, descriptions and definitions

Study type	Description	Definition
Observation	Diagnostic test evaluation	Definition of test sensitivity and specificity in experimental subgroups.
Observation	Meta-analysis	Studies in which the outcomes of multiple trials are combined. The power to identify significant results may be increased as very large numbers of subjects are included.
Observation	Systematic reviews	Structured analysis of the literature which is available on a particular topic. Methodologies to assess the relative values of different types of publication are in active development
Intervention	Experimental models	Studies which are conducted on an analogous system to the one of primary interest, e.g. leprosy in armadillos.
Intervention	Drug trials	Clinical trials where drugs are compared with placebo or alternative treatments allowing effectiveness to be assessed within or between groups of patients.
Intervention	*n* of 1 drug trials	A special case where a clinician assesses the effects of different treatments or treatment against placebo within an individual patient.
Intervention	Environment change	Studies when environmental factors are changed and outcomes observed in a form of intervention trial, e.g. campaigns to reduce smoking, increase road safety awareness, reduce lead in petrol.
Intervention	Clinical trials	Clinical trials where treatments (surgical, medical, physical) are compared with placebo or alternative treatments allowing effectiveness to be assessed within or between groups of patients.

Figure 4.2   Examples of study types, descriptions and definitions (continued)

Trial Type	Definition
Prospective studies	Studies in which data are collected in a planned manner over time. All intervention studies are prospective.
Retrospective studies	Studies where data are collected after the event for example from sets of pre-existing medical records.
Prospective analysis	Situations where data are collated against a predetermined set of criteria usually working towards an analytical end point which determines when data collection will cease.
Secondary analysis	Situations where previously collected data are subjected to secondary analysis to generate or prove new or extended hypotheses.
Cross-over studies	Studies in which the experimental subjects are exposed to one experimental condition in the first phase and are then changed to another condition in the second phase. This may or may not be in random order.
Single blind studies	Studies in which the subjects but not the experimenter are unaware of the conditions which are applied.
Double blind studies	Experiments in which neither the experimenter nor the subjects are informed of the treatment or control conditions to which they are assigned.
Phase 1 trials	Studies of basic pharmacology and toxicity. May be largely based on animal experimentation.
Phase 2 trials	Initial clinical investigations of efficacy and toxicity.
Phase 3 trials	Full scale clinical evaluation of therapeutic effectiveness.
Phase 4 trials	Postmarketing surveillance studies.
Meta-analysis	Analyses in which results of all relevant, independent and methodologically acceptable studies are combined.

Figure 4.3 Terms used to describe clinical trials

Two terms often used in the description of trials are *incidence* and *prevalence.* Incidence is the rate at which an event occurs over time; prevalence is the proportion of experimental subjects affected by a particular condition at a particular time.

Listed in Figure 4.4 are some classic trials drawn from the medical literature that indicate the historical origins of modern epidemiological studies. We have included two recent influential randomised control trials and a meta-analysis of the coronary thrombolytic intervention studies which would bear study.

Case control (retrospective) study

Smoking and carcinoma of the lung: preliminary report. Doll R, Hill A B. *Br Med J* 1950; **ii:** 739-48

Cohort (prospective) studies

The morbidity of doctors in relation to their smoking habits: a preliminary report. Doll R, Hill A B. *Br Med J* 1954; **i:** 1451-5

Lung cancer and other causes of death in relation to smoking: a second report on the morbidity of British doctors. Doll R, Hill A B. *Br Med J* 1956; **ii:** 1071-81

Randomised controlled trials

Streptomycin treatment of pulmonary tuberculosis: a Medical Research Council investigation. MRC Streptomycin in Tuberculosis Trials Committee. *Br Med J* 1948; **ii:** 769-82

Randomised trial of intravenous streptokinase, or aspirin, both, or neither among 17,187 cases of suspected myocardial infarction. ISIS-2 Collaborative Group. *Lancet* 1988; **ii:** 349-60

Randomised trial of cholesterol lowering in 4444 patients with coronary heart disease: the Scandinavian Simvastatin Survival Study (4S). The Scandinavian Simvastatin Survival Study Group. *Lancet* 1994; **344:** 1383-1389.

Meta-analysis

Effects of aspirin on coronary reocclusion and recurrent ischemia after thrombolysis: a meta-analysis. Roux S, Christeller S, Ludin E: *J Am Coll Cardiol 1992*; **19:** 671-677.

Figure 4.4 Some classic trials

WHY MAY SPECIAL STUDIES BE NEEDED FOR EVIDENCE-BASED MEDICINE AND CLINICAL AUDIT?

A recent trend in many countries has been to attempt to determine health policy on the basis of scientific evidence. In the UK this has been spearheaded by the NHS through its research and development initiative intended to ensure that medicine is practised on the basis of evidence rather than opinion (Culyer report, 1992).

WHAT IS MEANT BY EVIDENCE-BASED MEDICINE?

The basic premise is that many of the procedures conducted in routine practice have never been formally evaluated or subjected to scientific verification. Examples include topics as wide-ranging as laparoscopic surgery and physiotherapy. Furthermore, many procedures which have been scientifically verified as beneficial take several years to implement. An example of this would be the slow take-up of the use of aspirin therapy following myocardial infarction. The political imperative has therefore been to create health commissioning procedures which can be based on proven evidence. To underpin this a research programme has been formulated which incorporates four strands.

- Research to identify priorities in health care.
- The systematic use of reviews of published literature.
- Pro-active commissioning of rigorous research trials.
- The promotion and implementation of research findings.

The drive for such work comes from the widely held belief that the development of effective health care requires hard evidence, preferably from randomised trials, and that the use of such procedures either improves the natural history of disease or otherwise benefits patients at a reasonable cost (Cochrane, 1971/72). In assessing applied medical research it is necessary to take into account the underlying goal of a health system.

"The consensus wish to produce better health, defined as an improvement in the natural history of disease, in a manner which provides acceptable quality and at the same time provides value for money."

The criteria for evaluation of research used to formulate NHS policy can be categorised under the following headings:

Effectiveness -	does the procedure generate more health gain than the existing procedure?
Acceptability -	is the new procedure acceptable to patients and staff?
Efficiency -	does the new procedure generate more benefit per pound spent than an existing procedure?
The wider implications -	does the procedure affect other aspects of NHS activity or society in general?

It is clear that these extend far beyond narrow scientific boundaries and enter into areas of socio-political debate. They emphasise the social responsibility of science and challenge the ethics of adopting an amoral position on setting priorities for work based purely on scientific curiosity. Whether such a change of focus will inhibit innovation and reduce the possibility of serendipitous discoveries remains to be seen.

WHAT ARE THE DESIGN PROBLEMS OF EVIDENCE-BASED STUDIES?
One problem posed by the shift to evidence-based medicine is that classical scientific trials do not necessarily provide material which can answer the questions presented above. Though rigorous clinical trials may demonstrate that a procedure is more effective than an old procedure, it may not be able to answer questions such as whether efficiency is improved, nor necessarily whether the new procedure is more acceptable than the old procedure. In some cases classical randomised trial designs may be totally inappropriate for some of the assessments necessary in evidence-based medicine. For example, in some circumstances randomised trials may not be feasible because the controls necessary to account for value for money or effectiveness may be impossible to create. Furthermore the constraints imposed by the experimental design of a randomised trial may limit the ability to generalise the findings outside the experimental population, for example to other ethnic groups or to patients presenting via a different clinical service channel.

This is not to say that trials should be made less rigorous in order to meet the needs of evidence-based medicine or indeed that issues of randomisation can be bypassed. On the contrary, it is probably even more essential that care is taken to exclude bias in selection and analysis, since the intention to change practice on the basis of results is explicit. Schulz and colleagues have shown that trials which are poorly designed from the view of selection, blinding and randomisation give results which exaggerate the beneficial effects of treatment by as much as 41%. Furthermore, just because a trial claims to be randomised does not mean it was randomised appropriately and surveys of methodology show many deficiencies even in trials published in substantive journals.

A useful distinction which has been drawn is between trials which may be *explanatory*, that is, those designed along classical scientific lines and those which are *pragmatic* and which are designed to answer operational questions. Explanatory trials tend to be run under strict laboratory-style conditions using randomisation and controls, the aim being to increase the understanding of the underlying problem in terms of causation or effect. Pragmatic trials, on the other hand, may be utilised to make a choice between two procedures which are being used within normal clinical practice. They are generally created more along observation than intervention lines and work within the constraints and conditions prevailing in routine clinical practice. On face value these constraints usually mitigate against the adoption of classically controlled and randomised designs.

A number of other important differences exist between these two forms of trial which relate to differences in the approach to controls and the need to focus evaluation of outcome on a single composite measure of benefit and cost. Indeed, it is this latter aspect which presents the greatest challenge in relation to pragmatic trial design. The balance of cost and benefit must be weighed very carefully in creating the final composite measure if valid conclusions are to be reached. It has been suggested that the most effective treatment is the one which gives the better response on average as judged by the single comprehensive criterion. This may well not be amenable to statistical verification and providing a confidence interval for such a measure may be impossible. This then begs the question of how much better must a procedure be to warrant choosing over a rival? The answer may well be to trust to clinical and/or socio-political judgement.

It is worth pointing out that by its very nature the randomised, controlled trial lends itself to statistical analysis since the underlying assumption of statistical testing, randomisation, is inherent in the design. For pragmatic trials the fact that randomisation may not be explicit sometimes make it difficult to apply standard statistical procedures to the data. This is not to say that randomisation can be ignored, indeed the results of any trial, pragmatic or explanatory, which lack rigor in this regard should not be trusted.

To illustrate the possibilities for such pragmatic trials, consider the challenge of evaluating a surgical procedure such as radical prostatectomy for prostate cancer. In the first place, such trials cannot be placebo-controlled as there is no verifiable placebo which could be ethically utilised. The trials similarly cannot operate on a double-blind basis. It is difficult to randomise the recruitment of patients for a treatment or no treatment option, since the participating surgeons are likely to have quite strong prejudices for or against such a procedure, which will itself determine their referral patterns and bias patient selection. In addition, it is difficult to control the surgical skill levels between centres and similarly to allow for patient prejudices and preferences which will again distort referral patterns.

Surgical trials often compare new procedures against long established ones and there will be a learning curve effect. This may occur in two ways. Firstly, inexperienced surgeons will be learning the new procedures in the initial stages and the outcomes are likely to be poorer. Secondly, trials may be biased because the innovators may actually have more native skill than the general surgical population. Though many of these objections will undermine a fully randomised double-blind trial, if viewed in the context of a pragmatic trial all variables such as referral patterns or patient preference need legitimate evaluation. The absence of placebos may not be important if the procedures under review are realistic choices for the health commissioners. Placebo effects may actually be beneficial if patient well-being improves. Equally, the lack of randomisation and double-blindness at the outset of the trial may be of no importance if the trial evaluation is carried out in a blind, or at least an unbiased, fashion.

Methods which can be employed to construct such pragmatic trials include the creation of multicentre trials to increase numbers and smooth out the effects of patient selection or surgical skill, or the employment of a method of analysis which compares the data of several single-centre trials of each of the procedures in a pragmatic manner. Specific methods may be undertaken to control patient preferences using trials which apply randomisation to patients who are indifferent between the choice of procedures, or randomised consent trials where patients are randomised only after they have consented. Other aspects, such as the effects of learning curves and differences in skill levels, can be overcome by running extended trials or actively monitoring the performance of doctors over time. A trial which illustrates some of these approaches is included in the bibliography (Wasson *et al*, 1995).

A similar challenge can be made concerning the introduction of new drugs into clinical practice. Double-blind placebo-controlled trials can certainly establish the effectiveness of a new drug. The pragmatic question, however, is whether the new drug is better or worse than an established drug. Studies to answer such questions may be difficult to mount in a double-blind manner. For example, if a once-a-day drug preparation is compared with a many times a day preparation it will be difficult to run this study double-blind without resorting to complex double-dummy designs. There is the potential that the more frequently taken drug may actually have a bigger placebo effect than the once-a-day drug. In an explanatory trial interested in efficacy but not convenience this can be controlled by instituting the use of a dummy ineffective agent, on an equal number of occasions. If a pragmatic approach is taken, the requirement is to assess the overall outcome and the placebo effect will be included in the outcome. In order to analyse for this a more complex design which includes controls for once-a-day use may be required. If placebo effects play an important part in the clinical process under review then this needs to be appropriately weighed in the final decision concerning which treatment to adopt.

In summary, the development of research methodologies suitable for evidence-based medicine is a considerable challenge which will require careful appraisal of the outcome measures and their evaluation if respectable conclusions are to be drawn.

IS CLINICAL AUDIT THE SAME AS CLINICAL RESEARCH?

The principal function of clinical audit is to enhance the quality of clinical service delivery. It does this by attempting to ensure that practice adheres to defined policies or procedures which have been identified as those most likely to produce the best results. In the future audit may well become the major local effector mechanism for evidence-based medicine, but at present the focus tends to be confined to assessment of the pragmatic issues of service delivery. Although clinical audit may utilise research techniques it has more in common with the Continuous Quality Improvement (CQI) approach to quality management than to scientific research *per se.*

Audit activity is generally held to be cyclical in nature and four distinct phases can be identified.

- *Phase 1* is concerned with identifying the standards which constitute best practice.
- In *Phase 2* these standards are constituted into a policy or procedure against which performance can be assessed.
- In *Phase 3* current practice is assessed to determine whether the policy or procedures are adhered to.
- *Phase 4* is a stage of review when either current practice and/or the policy or procedure is updated in the light of the actual findings.

Audit could be viewed as analogous to the derivation and testing of a scientific hypothesis but in practice audit differs considerably from scientific research. Control conditions are rarely employed and blinding and randomisation techniques are often not feasible in this context. However, issues such as whether changes are significant, reproducible or transferable are still relevant and the adoption of appropriate best practice techniques drawn from scientific experimentation can still be of great value. Sloppy or biased data collection will undermine any conclusions drawn in an audit process and such conclusions could prove extremely dangerous especially if used directly to change a clinical procedure or policy.

One should not conclude that audit simply constitutes poor research. Like evidence-based medicine, clinical audit throws up many significant challenges in terms of study design and analysis. The critical point is again to understand the fundamental basis of the questions being asked and then to apply scientific methods appropriately where these are suitable and/or necessary.

This section has outlined the terminology used in the field of clinical experimentation and has provided an introduction to some of the issues involved in trial design. Much can be gained by learning to assess trial designs critically as flaws in the design of trials can crucially undermine the validity of conclusions which can be drawn. Such an understanding can be helpful in developing a healthy scepticism as far as adopting practices promoted on the basis of clinical trials. Also many pitfalls of trial design can be avoided by building on knowledge gained in this way.

HOW SHOULD A STUDY BE RUN?

Running studies whether big or small is not a simple task. High levels of commitment and motivation are essential and are often needed to counter the frustrations encountered as studies unfold. Research is a highly individualised process. Trials are usually unique events and consequently can take lots of effort for a small, one-off return. The glamorous view of the Nobel prize-winning 'Eureka-style' discoveries are seldom, if ever, met - hard grind for what, in 99% of cases, may be no more than a small scientific advance, a couple of citations and a little reflected glory is the watchword. Young clinicians often fail to realise that although science lacks the drama of clinical practice, as a professional activity it is no less exacting and requires just as much hard won practical experience for success.

The major goal of research must be to influence practice, either of one's own or that of one's peers, even if on occasion the change in practice is simply to identify the need for more research. Publication plays a crucial part in this process. After all, if you discover something worthwhile you will wish others to know the fact and to add it to the body of shared scientific knowledge. Therefore it is essential to consider any experimental plan in relation to how you will eventually communicate the answers.

A recent trend in papers has been to develop structured abstracts such as the one shown in Figure 4.5. Note the clear definition of the problem, the description of the study design, the subjects employed and the data gathered, the clear presentation of the results and the concluding discussion of the interpretation of the findings. This structure will be used for the rest of the discussion which will present a project management approach to study design and execution.

PROJECT MANAGEMENT

Embarking on a research project with the hope that something will turn up is a recipe for frustration and disappointment. Meticulous planning and execution are just as important as good analytical technique.

Industry has developed schemes of project management and we would recommend this approach in defining and running any study. Project management essentially involves breaking the process down into a series of achievable steps, considering what needs to be done to complete each and analysing any contingencies between stages so that the sequence can be properly maintained. It is very useful as a means of foreseeing difficulties which could arise and therefore planning to avoid them.

Effect on lipoprotein profile of replacing butter with margarine in a low fat diet: randomised crossover study with hypercholesterolaemic subjects

A Chisholm, J Mann, W Sutherland *et al*   *Br Med J* 1996; **312**: 931-4

Objective – To examine the effect on lipid and lipoprotein concentrations when butter or an unsaturated margarine is used for cooking or spreading in a reduced fat diet.

Design – Randomised crossover study with two intervention periods of six weeks' duration separated by a five week washout.

Setting – Community setting in New Zealand.

Subjects – 49 volunteers with polygenic hypercholesterolaemia and baseline cholesterol in the range 5.5 - 7.9 mmol/L.

Main outcome measures – Concentrations of total and low density lipoprotein, Lp(a) lipoprotein, high density lipoprotein, apolipoprotein B 100, and apolipoprotein A I.

Results – Concentrations of low density lipoprotein cholesterol and apolipoprotein B were about 10% lower with margarine than with butter. Lp(a) lipoprotein and high density lipoprotein cholesterol concentrations were similar with the two diets.

Conclusion – Despite concerns about adverse effects on lipoproteins of *trans* fatty acids in margarines, the use of unsaturated margarine rather than butter in hypercholesterolaemic people is associated with a lipoprotein profile that would be expected to reduce cardiovascular disease.

Figure 4.5   Example of a structured abstract

At first glance project management may appear to be no more than merely the application of a little common sense. However, it is worth spending time on the basics as it provides some very useful tools for the planning and execution phases. Sufficient of the rudiments can be picked up with minimal study though the subject can become extremely complex, for example if applied to large scale projects or multicentre projects. A useful book on the subject is *Project Management: from idea to implementation* by Haynes which can be read cover to cover in little over an hour.

In simple terms any study would fall into stages of: a) Planning, b) Execution and c) Reporting, assuming that the essential first step of identifying a research goal has already been achieved. Each stage can be broken into sub-components as shown in Figure 4.6.

Phase of project	Activities
Planning	Clarifying the objectives Conducting a thorough literature review Generating / modifying the hypothesis Designing the study Defining the protocol Gaining ethical approval Identifying the resources (people, equipment, methods, money)
Execution	Recruiting the subjects Initiating the investigation Collecting the data Analysing the data
Reporting	Presenting the data Preparing the report / paper Submitting for publication Modifying in the light of referees' comments.

Figure 4.6   An outline project plan

A useful tool is the Gantt chart which allows the time sequence and contingencies between stages to be readily visualised. An example is given in Figure 4.7. Each stage should have a definite end point, referred to as a milestone, and these can be monitored to assess progress. Failure to achieve such a milestone can be used to determine whether progress is satisfactory and whether corrective action is necessary. Some stages of a project may be iterative and a milestone check can be set such that a particular stage is repeated if necessary. For example, if the literature review indicated that part of the underlying question had been answered or provided evidence that the objectives were inappropriate then returning to the objective setting stage would be necessary. Though this can clearly be a dispiriting event a well-honed project is more likely to be successful. It is better to pull back early rather than commit precious resources to fruitless activity.

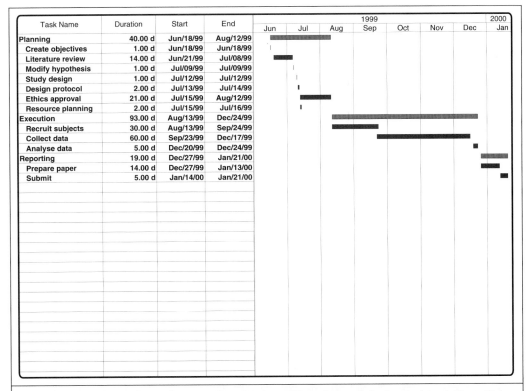

Task Name	Duration	Start	End
Planning	40.00 d	Jun/18/99	Aug/12/99
Create objectives	1.00 d	Jun/18/99	Jun/18/99
Literature review	14.00 d	Jun/21/99	Jul/08/99
Modify hypothesis	1.00 d	Jul/09/99	Jul/09/99
Study design	1.00 d	Jul/12/99	Jul/12/99
Design protocol	2.00 d	Jul/13/99	Jul/14/99
Ethics approval	21.00 d	Jul/15/99	Aug/12/99
Resource planning	2.00 d	Jul/15/99	Jul/16/99
Execution	93.00 d	Aug/13/99	Dec/24/99
Recruit subjects	30.00 d	Aug/13/99	Sep/24/99
Collect data	60.00 d	Sep/23/99	Dec/17/99
Analyse data	5.00 d	Dec/20/99	Dec/24/99
Reporting	19.00 d	Dec/27/99	Jan/21/00
Prepare paper	14.00 d	Dec/27/99	Jan/13/00
Submit	5.00 d	Jan/14/00	Jan/21/00

This figure shows the Gantt chart used to manage an imaginary clinical experiment. By outlining each stage of a study and assigning times and contingencies between them an overall picture of the study can be obtained. Note that in some cases the processes overlap and in others are arranged sequentially. A Gantt chart is a useful planning tool for calculating how much time a project will take to complete and is also useful for tracking performance as progress can be plotted on the chart and slippage identified. For the historically minded, H L Gantt described his chart for use solving scheduling problems in 1917.

Figure 4.7 Project management Gantt chart

It is good practice to document the project as it develops. A useful scheme is to create a booklet describing the project and to maintain this as the master plan. For guidance the contents page of the protocol for an imaginary MRC trial on prostate cancer is shown in Figure 4.8. The headings in such a document are largely self-explanatory. The sections which follow indicate how such a document can be developed and put into practice. Remember as you put the document together that it will undergo scrutiny by many of your peers. It is worth imagining yourself in this position working down a checklist of criteria by which you would evaluate the proposal. If you cannot pass your own scrutiny then more work is needed! (See section on How to Evaluate a Proposal, page 160)

The ALCAP Trial is a double blind, placebo controlled trial of the use of antileukin for control of bone metastases in carcinoma of the prostate. A published protocol for such a trial would be expected to include the following sections:

1.	Trial outline
2.	Objectives
		Primary objective
		Secondary objectives
3.	Background
4.	Patient selection
		Eligibility criteria
		Ethical considerations
5.	Randomisation
6.	Supply of drugs
7.	Pretreatment and on-study investigations
		Examinations required before entry
		Studies during treatment
		Recommended investigations
		Mandatory investigations
8.	Drug administration
9.	Dose modifications
		Gastro-intestinal upset
		Renal function impairment
		Allergic reactions
		Haematological disturbances
10.	Adverse events / Adverse drug reactions
11.	Follow-up
		One month tolerability check
		Maintenance
		First symptomatic bone progression or death
12.	Statistical considerations
		Trial size
		Interim analysis
		Data monitoring committee
13.	Progress reports
14.	Additional evaluations on trial patients
15.	Publication
16.	References

Appendices
- TNM Classification
- WHO performance status
- Data collection documentation
- Adverse events
- Patient information sheet
- Patient consent form

Figure 4.8   An example study protocol

PLANNING

Getting planning right prevents later disappointment and difficulties. No amount of sophisticated statistical analysis can salvage a badly designed or executed study.

DEFINING /REDEFINING THE QUESTION (EXPERIMENTAL HYPOTHESIS)

This is probably the most important stage of all, since if the question is properly posed at the outset all else should follow logically in its wake. The popular view that scientists 'discover' things through some kind of inspirational magic is totally fallacious. A novel idea may be based on an insight that an observation does not make sense, or that there is possibly a better way of doing something, but taking the steps to knowing what to do or how to prove it are cold calculated decisions.

Question	Possible experimental hypothesis to test
Does preoperative testing of urea and electrolytes prevent the occurrence of complications?	Patients in whom pre-operative tests were carried out have a lower complication rate than in matched patients in whom no tests were done.
Is recurrent otitis media the result of immunodeficiency?	The prevalence of immunodeficiency is higher in patients with otitis media than it is in an age-matched control group.
Is a fasting sample needed for reliable estimation of lipid status?	Fasting samples have lower concentrations of cholesterol and triglycerides than samples drawn from the same patients post-prandially.
Do servicemen from the Gulf War suffer from an unexpectedly high risk of debilitating illness?	The incidence of non-specific wasting disease is higher in Gulf War veterans than in controls matched for age, gender, exposure to foreign travel and social status.
Does adjuvant chemotherapy prevent recurrence of resectable oesophageal cancer?	The survival of patients with operable oesophageal cancer given peri-operative chemotherapy is longer than those given no chemotherapy.

Figure 4.9   Some possible questions and experimental hypotheses

Notice that the hypotheses listed are effectively binary statements which should give a clear true or false answer. They necessarily beg a number of questions which require development such as "How does one define suitable experimental and control groups?" or, for example, "What constitutes the difference between a fasting and a post-prandial sample?" It is through iterative consideration of the study design that such questions are identified and clarified. Also, in these examples we have identified only one hypothesis per question. Several parallel hypotheses may be evident and it may be necessary to rank these in order of importance and to consider whether it is practical to study them simultaneously, or whether separate studies or trials would be needed. In the last example although survival is an important end point, it may be of interest to consider whether quality of life is or is not affected by the use of chemotherapy. Thus a secondary hypothesis might be that irrespective of survival, the quality of life of the patients is poorer in the group treated with chemotherapy because of the associated morbidity due to side-effects of the drugs.

A good exercise for improving skills is to take a dozen or so papers and try to:

- identify the primary scientific or clinical question
- assess whether an appropriate hypothesis was generated
- review how the hypothesis was tested
- consider whether the original question was answered

In a random selection of papers even from high quality journals there will be times when it will be difficult to conclude that all four stages have been adequately completed. As an extension to the exercise, reviewing the correspondence about a paper can be helpful in identifying deficiencies or controversial points. Indeed the correspondence pages of journals provide an excellent site for public scrutiny and act as a final court of appeal where conflicting views about the scientific quality of information can be fought out.

REVIEWING THE LITERATURE

The next logical step is to undertake a formal review of literature. It is likely that in considering the question for investigation background literature will have been considered. However, it is worth stepping back at this stage and re-reviewing the available literature. The essential issue with the literature review is that it should be timely, of sufficient breadth to cover all the major issues and should be conducted in sufficient depth to ensure that the development of the protocol and experimental plan do not contain serious avoidable flaws. Given the volume of published data that exists in medicine (303,070 papers were indexed on Medline in 1995) this is not a trivial task, and a balance has to be struck between a comprehensive review and an effective survey of available information. The important issue is to identify the seminal papers on a topic and to extract the central themes. It is essential that a well balanced view of the material under study is developed. It is easy to fall into the trap of biasing a review towards a favoured hypothesis and in this way to undermine the value of the whole project. An important skill is the ability to identify when it is necessary to refer to detail within the published material rather than to rely upon information in review articles or editorials.

REFINING THE HYPOTHESIS

Having defined the question the next step is to work out logically what is needed to answer it. One might work out hypothetically what conclusion might be drawn from each possible outcome and consider whether such an answer or outcome would be of value.

DEFINING THE PROTOCOL

Having decided on a question and formulated the null hypothesis, the next step is to work out the experimental protocol which can provide the evidence to prove or refute the hypothesis. This is not as easy as it sounds. It is quite possible to pose a significant question, to identify an hypothesis and then to realise that it is actually impossible to define an experimental protocol capable of providing the necessary evidence. This may be for ethical, financial or technical reasons. Where this happens it may be necessary to return to the question, or to recognise that, for example, a stage of methodological development is needed before proceeding with the main project.

DEFINING THE STUDY GROUP(S)

This can be easy in some cases but is often a point of severe contention. Careful selection of appropriate patient groups or experimental material can help to improve the power of an experiment to reach the appropriate conclusion. Though this may appear to be biased in the direction of favourable outcomes, on occasion the selection of inappropriate groups may mask a real effect or difference. The inclusion of excessive random noise can be as undesirable as inappropriate over-selection of subjects.

DECIDING HOW TO AVOID BIAS USING RANDOMISATION

The first question here is whether randomisation is necessary. In most cases the answer will be "yes" as randomisation plays a pivotal role in preventing false results through selection bias. Even in an experiment to compare the results of measuring the same substance using two methods on the same sample it may be necessary to consider randomisation of testing in order to eliminate errors introduced by carryover, decay of the substance under test etc. Similarly, though randomisation is not usually applied formally, in observational studies and surveys it is essential to ensure that methods of patient selection are not subject to systematic error which would invalidate any conclusions.

Patients, experimental animals or laboratory specimens can be allocated to one of two groups by the toss of a coin, or by using the sequence of odd and even numbers either provided in a table of random numbers or generated by a computer's random number generator. Random numbers can also be used for allocation to more than two groups - for example, by using 1, 2 and 3 for the first group, 4, 5 and 6 for the second and 7, 8 and 9 for the third, ignoring values of 0.

To make sure that the numbers of subjects allocated to each group remain closely matched, a scheme of *block allocation* can be used. If there are two groups, x and y, then there are six possible sequences for blocks of four subjects, two of each group in each block of four (xxyy, xyxy, xyyx, yyxx, yxyx and yxxy). These blocks are given numbers from 1 to 6 and random numbers, ignoring values of 7, 8, 9 and 0, are used to decide the order in which groups are allocated. Using this system the numbers in the two groups can differ by only two at the most. An analogous method can be used for more than two groups. The investigator should be unaware of the method of randomization because the last allocation in each block can be deduced from the earlier allocations.

Stratified block randomization is used if it is important to match specific characteristics of the members of the groups, for example, sex and smoking history. In this case it is necessary to use a separate block allocation list for each combination of characteristics, in the example, male smokers, female smokers, male non-smokers and female non-smokers. Similarly, stratification by different ranges of a variable can be used to ensure that groups of patients have a similar age distribution or similar cholesterol concentrations, or that groups of experimental animals are of similar weight.

An acceptable alternative to stratified block randomization, particularly in small clinical trials, is to use *minimization*. Essentially this consists of allocating the next patient to enter the trial to the treatment group where his or her combination of characteristics will minimize the differences between the characteristics of the patients already in the groups. For more detailed discussion, see Akazawa *et al* and Pocock (see Further Reading).

CHOOSING APPROPRIATE STATISTICAL TESTS

Having decided what is going to be measured and what outcome is required to test the null hypothesis, an appropriate statistical test should be chosen. The following steps will guide readers through the table of commonly used tests and in the majority of cases will lead to the correct choice of test.

1. Consider what type of data you are dealing with (classified, ranked or measured) since this is a major determinant of which tests can be used.

2. Consider what sort of difference, change or association might be observed. In particular, decide whether the predicted change or difference will be uni-directional or in either direction. From this decide whether a one- or two-tailed test of significance will be needed. (Be prepared to justify the choice of a one-tailed test.)

3. Assess whether the underlying assumptions of the statistical test will be met by the data, for example whether the data should be Normally distributed.

4. If, from your knowledge of the subject area, the assumptions are not met consider whether data transformation will allow them to be met.

5. If it is not possible to meet the assumptions of the first choice test then it may be necessary to choose an alternative test. This is common in the case of measured data where non-parametric tests can often be used as alternatives. Parametric tests cannot be used as alternatives for ranked data.

6. If necessary, estimate the numbers of subjects needed to achieve the required level of statistical significance (page 150).

For example, consider the data analysis for a 'before and after' treatment study. The data will be in the form of measured values. The design is naturally a paired comparison and the null hypothesis is that there will be no difference between the results measured before and after treatment. Thus, a paired t-test would be an appropriate test here.

The assumption is that the distribution of differences will be Normal and this distribution should be visualised with a Normal probability plot (page 11) before conducting the analysis. If it is not Normal then a transformation may need to be applied. If this fails to Normalise the values then a Wilcoxon matched-pairs test might be used (page 62).

As can be seen, the form of the data may be visible only when the experiment itself has been conducted and on many occasions one has to make best guess judgements. In large projects this may be unacceptable if large amounts of time, effort and money are to be committed to the experiment. If this state of affairs is reached then it is often worth going back a stage and running a pilot experiment to answer as many of the uncertainties as possible, otherwise large amounts of effort may be expended to little purpose.

HOW DOES ONE CHOOSE AN APPROPRIATE STATISTICAL TEST?

Listed below are the tests that can be applied to different types of classified, ranked and measured data together with the null hypothesis that is tested. The heading 'Requirements' lists some of the limiting criteria. The requirement for a Normal distribution for the tests listed under measured data can sometimes be fulfilled by transformation, usually logarithmic (page 16). The alternative tests listed for measured data are not distribution dependent (non-parametric). The advantages and disadvantages of least squares linear regression, Deming regression and Passing and Bablok regression for describing a linear relationship between two groups of measured data are discussed in Chapter 2 (page 54).

Type of data	Null hypothesis	Test	Requirements	Alternative test
Two by two table of independent frequencies	No association between rows and columns	Fisher's exact test (page 6)	Good computer hardware and software if frequencies large, no lower limit	Chi-squared (χ^2) test
Two by two or larger table of independent frequencies	No association between rows and columns	χ^2 test with continuity correction (page 61)	80% of expected frequencies greater than 5, none 0 or 1	Fisher's exact test if 2x 2 or merge classes
Two by two table of paired frequencies	No difference, so equal frequencies in the two discordant cells	McNemar's χ^2 test with continuity correction (page 60)	Sum of discordant pairs at least 10	Exact binomial probability (see Kirkwood)

Figure 4.10   Tests for classified data

Type of data	Null hypothesis	Test	Requirements	Alternative test
Two groups of independent ranked data	Groups are samples from the same population	Mann-Whitney U-test corrected for ties (page 8)	None	Wilcoxon's rank sum T-test gives the same probability value
More than two groups of independent ranked data	Groups are samples from the same population	Kruskal-Wallis one-way analysis of variance corrected for ties	None	None
Two groups of paired ranked data	Paired ranks do not differ	Wilcoxon matched-pairs signed-ranks test corrected for ties (page 62)	None	None
Two groups of paired ranked data	Paired ranks are not associated	Spearman rank correlation corrected for ties	None	Kendall rank correlation is an equally powerful alternative

Figure 4.11   Tests on ranked data or non-Normal measured data

Type of data	Null hypothesis	Test	Requirements	Alternative test
A single group of independent measured data	Group mean does not differ from a specified value	One sample t-test (page 38)	Normal distribution	None
Two groups of independent measured data	Groups are samples from the same Normal population	F-test for variances (page 31)	Normal distributions	None
Two small groups of independent measured data	Groups are samples from the same Normal population	Two sample t-test for means of small samples (page 41)	Normal distributions Similar variances	Mann-Whitney U-test
Two large groups of independent measured data	Groups are samples from the same Normal population	Two sample t-test for means of large samples (page 40)	Normal distributions Variances may be unequal	Mann-Whitney U-test
More than two groups of independent measured data	Groups are samples from the same Normal population	One-way analysis of variance (page 33)	Normal distributions Similar variances	Kruskal-Wallis one-way analysis of variance
Two groups of paired measured data	Mean difference is zero	Paired t-test (page 59)	Normal distribution of differences	Wilcoxon matched-pairs signed-ranks test corrected for ties
Two groups of paired measured data	No linear relationship between variables	Pearson correlation	Normal distributions	Spearman or Kendall rank correlation

Figure 4.12 Tests on measured data

ESTIMATING THE NUMBERS OF SUBJECTS NEEDED

Having decided on the test which is likely to be used, it is then possible to proceed to estimate the number of subjects that should be included to test the null hypothesis reliably. It is a frequent finding in medical research that the size of a trial is well below that necessary to provide a definitive answer to the question being asked. This is such a problem that grant-giving bodies currently insist that researchers carry out power calculations to estimate the subject numbers needed. Power calculations may appear complex but in reality are quite straightforward.

Suppose we wish to know whether delays in sample transport affect glucose values measured in the laboratory. Such might be the case, for example, when considering routine screening samples transported into the laboratory from general practice sites compared with those collected within the hospital outpatient clinic. Our research hypothesis is that GP samples have lower average glucose concentrations than samples obtained in outpatients. At the outset the reliability of the analytical techniques is usually known, as well as both the size of a clinically important difference between the two situations under investigation and the rough spread of values expected within the samples obtained. We will assume that the populations screened are similar and known diabetic patients have been excluded. The data could be expected to fall into the form shown in Figure 4.13.

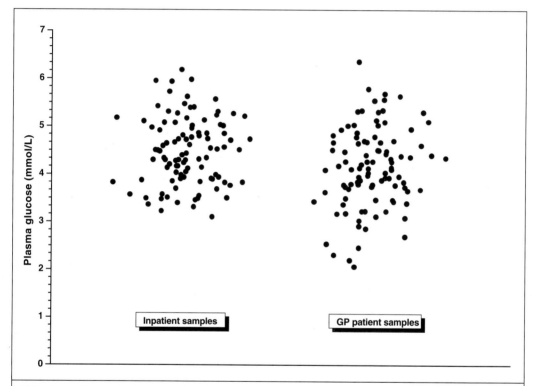

This shows the preliminary results obtained in a comparison of glucose measurements made on samples received from general practice and from in-patients. There is an impression that the GP samples are somewhat lower than the in-patient samples, though they have a wider variance. The question is to decide how many samples should be measured to show with confidence that the difference is real.

Figure 4.13 Estimating sample sizes

As seen earlier, we can improve our confidence in the reliability of derived parameters by increasing the number of subjects measured. In this case, increasing the numbers in the groups will improve our confidence in the estimates of the true means of the populations and, thereby, increase our ability to discriminate between them. This is shown graphically in Figure 4.14. As the numbers increase the overlap between the estimates of the true means (shown in the lower panels) of the two measurements is reduced to the point where they are clearly separated.

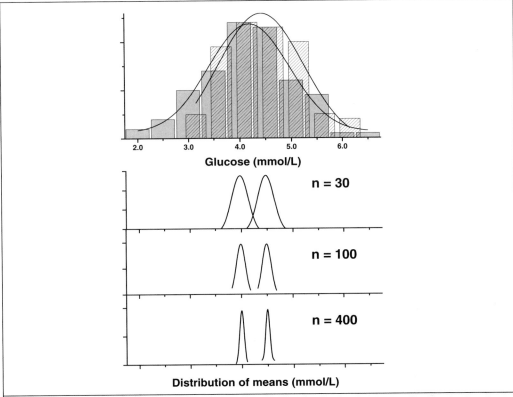

This figure demonstrates the importance of subject numbers in increasing the confidence in concluding whether two samples are drawn from the same or different populations. In the upper panel the data from Figure 4.13 is redrawn as histograms with overlaid distribution profiles. The impression is again that the specimens from the GPs give lower glucose values than those from the hospital patients. In the lower panels are shown the distributions for the means ± the standard errors of the means for the two samples for fixed values of mean and SD. As the number of observations in the samples is increased, the standard error diminishes and though the means stay static the degree of overlap of the distributions of the means is reduced. As the overlap reduces so confidence that the difference is real increases. By working out the n which would produce the appropriate degree of overlap for a given degree of confidence in the result it is possible to estimate the sample numbers needed. This principle applies to all situations where estimates of numbers are needed. Increasing the numbers of subjects produces tighter confidence ranges and therefore more robust discrimination.

Figure 4.14   Estimating sample sizes

To translate this into a calculation of required numbers we need to be aware of two factors. The first is the confidence we can have in our estimates of the population means which increases with the numbers used. The second is the magnitude of the minimal difference between the groups which, if present, we accept as showing the groups to be truly distinct. Setting this requires judgement as to what represents a true clinically significant difference. We could, for example, accept a small minimal difference but then might merely prove that a difference existed that was of no clinical relevance. Alternatively, making the minimal difference too large might be inadvisable because if it is beyond clinical feasibility the hypothesis may be falsely rejected.

These two factors interact. If the minimal difference is small, numbers must be large to provide the precision necessary for the discrimination. Numbers will be smaller for the same level of analytical imprecision if the minimal difference is larger but clinical feasibility might be exceeded.

CALCULATING REQUIRED 'N'

Two statistical concepts are relevant to calculating numbers required which relate to the reliability of the outcome of the statistical evaluation. They are the statistical significance of the result and the power of the test. These are defined as:

Statistical significance	The maximum probability that the null hypothesis under test is falsely rejected when it is in fact true (Type 1 error) is commonly referred to as **alpha**. The statistical significance is **alpha** expressed as a percentage.
Power	The maximum accepted probability of failing to reject the null hypothesis when it is actually untrue (Type 2 error) is commonly referred to as **beta**. The power of a test is calculated as (1 - **beta**). It is usually expressed as a percentage.

Figure 4.15 Statistical significance and power

The exact values chosen for alpha and beta depend on the scientific or clinical costs involved in reaching an inappropriate conclusion. Setting too high a threshold of acceptance will make it impossible to carry out the experiment, whilst setting too low a threshold increases the risk of reaching false conclusions and thus of the consequences in terms of morbidity, mortality and wasted resources. Typically alpha and beta are set asymmetrically. A 5% chance of wrongly accepting the null hypothesis (*alpha = 0.05*) is commonly used, whereas values for failing to reject an untrue hypotheses are more likely to be in the range 10 - 20% (*beta = 0.10 to 0.20*), that is, a power of 80-90%. These figures thus reflect the relative costs of reaching false positive or false negative conclusions and may need modification depending upon the exact nature of the clinical trial and the likely significance of the results. Higher thresholds may be set in assessing whether the adoption of a mass screening programme for cancer is justified than in selecting which test to use to diagnose hypothyroidism. Assessing the threshold for acceptable risk is a science in itself and is not as simple as it might appear at first sight. Those with an interest in this area are recommended to read Kirkwood's book.

When values for alpha and beta have been chosen, it is possible to calculate the numbers required in any experiment to reach the desired confidence levels. For our example, suppose it was suspected that the delay in separation of samples from GP patients would lower plasma glucose measurements by at least 0.5 mmol/L. A suitable design would be to compare the mean results of GP patient samples against a similar set collected in the outpatient clinic. The design is thus an unpaired comparison of two sets of data and the test is against a null hypothesis that there would be no difference or that the outpatients would have lower values. Since the direction of change is predicted a one-sided test of significance is appropriate. The distributions of samples are expected to lie within the reference range of plasma glucose (3.0 - 6.0 mmol/L) giving an SD of approximately 0.75 mmol/L for the two groups. If the experimenter were looking to reliably detect a reduction of around 0.5 mmol/L with a power of 80% at the 5% level then at least 28 subjects in each group would be necessary. It is important to emphasise that the threshold difference is the smallest difference we want to be able to detect reliably and is not necessarily equal to the expected difference. If the threshold difference were made smaller, say 0.2 mmol/L, then it would be necessary to include as many as 174 samples from each group to test this statistically.

FORMULAE FOR SAMPLE SIZE CALCULATIONS
Similar calculations can be made for any number of experimental designs. In Figure 4.16 are the formulae which can be applied for commonly used experimental protocols where measured Normally distributed data are obtained. Formulae for situations where classified or ranked data is considered are more complex and can be found in Kirkwood's book.

Some software packages provide facilities to carry out these calculations once the appropriate estimates are entered. It is important to select the correct model in order to reach acceptable conclusions.

The following sequence should be followed in estimating sample sizes:

1. Decide what model the experiment approximates to.

2. For tests seeking a significant difference decide:

    • the required level of significance (typically 0.05 or 5%)

    • the size of the minimum difference between the mean and a hypothetical value or between the population means

    • the required test power (typically 0.8 or 80%)

Follow the calculations in Figure 4.16 where:

a is the percentage point of the Normal distribution corresponding to the required significance level of the experiment, i.e. *alpha x 100*. For 5% significance this is 1.96.

b is the percentage point of the Normal distribution corresponding to (100 - the required power of the experiment), i.e. *beta x 100*. For 80% power this is 1.28.

SD, SDx and **SDy** are the expected SDs of the samples.

Comparison of a single mean against a hypothetical value	$\dfrac{(a + b)^2 \times SD^2}{(mean - value)^2}$
Comparison of two means (numbers required in each group)	$\dfrac{(a + b)^2 \times (SD_x^2 + SD_y^2)}{(mean_x - mean_y)^2}$

Figure 4.16 Calculation of the numbers required to reach significance

3. For tests seeking a particular degree of precision decide:

    • the required degree of precision

    • identify the expected SD(s) of the mean(s) of interest

Follow the calculation in Figure 4.17 where :

SE is the required SE of a single mean or of the difference between two means

SD, SD$_x$ and **SD$_y$** are the expected SDs of the samples.

For a single mean	$$\dfrac{SD^2}{SE^2}$$
For the difference between two means	$$\dfrac{SD_x^2 + SD_y^2}{SE^2}$$

Figure 4.17 Calculation of numbers required to reach a desired level of precision

OBTAINING ETHICAL APPROVAL

The basic ethical question is whether the risks to the patient of the work can be justified by the potential benefits. This can be a vexed question and proof or refutation of the argument may demand much of the effort of developing the study in the first place.

Most local Ethics Committees will issue guidelines on what studies require ethical approval and how this should be carried out. Ethical considerations for human studies are based on the Helsinki Declaration (1975) which has been adopted globally as the yardstick for clinical trials. It is best to err on the side of caution and submit any study involving patients, human volunteers or human material for ethical approval. If it is unnecessary the local committee will say so. Animal experimentation is also subject to strict controls, by the Home Office in the UK, as is embryological (Human Embryo and Fertilisation Authority) and genetic research.

There are many instances where seemingly straightforward routine laboratory studies throw up unexpected ethical problems. For example, using surplus routine clinical material to establish reference ranges, though accepted practice, can lead to dilemmas if unexpected abnormal results are identified. Is it the duty of the laboratory scientist to report such a finding to the patient's physician or to the patient themselves or to ignore it? Similarly, if such material is used for method development, what is the position if such work involves commercial support or sponsorship? It should be remembered that the sale of human material is forbidden and all patient data must be treated as strictly confidential. Routine material will not have been obtained with informed consent for extra scientific procedures. With proper planning these problems should be anticipated at the outset. Clearly, there is a common sense position which suggests that this routine work is necessary and would be fatally inhibited were all such studies subject to the full rigours of clinical trial regulation. However it is better to be proactive and seek approval openly at the outset, than to suffer potential embarrassment and even litigation or prosecution should the unexpected occur.

At a practical level the issue of informed consent can raise many problems. There has been a vigorous debate of this matter in relation to clinical practice and the problem becomes more difficult in the area of research. Where new treatments are concerned it may be that patients will be unable to make an informed choice as the evidence is simply unavailable. Special measures may be necessary to ensure that consent is fairly obtained, possibly by someone who is not attached to the investigation team. For a detailed examination of the issue the reader is encouraged to read one of the newer texts on medical ethics e.g. that from the BMA.

Shown below are examples of a consent form and a patient information sheet modelled on ones used in an actual trial. These can be taken as models on which to develop ones suitable for new trials. Patient information sheets ensure that patients are better informed about the nature of proposed research than has been usual in the past when consent was often obtained verbally. Analysis of patient's understanding of what they had agreed to, has shown that they were ill-informed in many cases and might have refused consent had they been given written information. However, it should not be felt that formal information sheets necessarily make patients more likely to refuse consent as such sheets can increase thier confidence in the value of the work to be undertaken and increase their willingness to participate.

SEEKING FUNDING

Seeking funding for a study or trial can be a disheartening experience. The restrictions on funding for research coupled with the ever increasing demand makes this an extremely competitive process. The average success rate for applications lies between 1 in 5 and 1 in 10 so be prepared to submit a lot proposals and to receive a lot of rejections! It is worth considering that as much work goes into a small application as a large one and it may be better to submit a few high quality large grants than several of lower value. There are many sources of funding some general, such as the MRC, and some highly specific where the funds are earmarked for a particular purpose, e.g. the BMA awards which are often supported by legacies left for particular purposes. Increasingly, even general funds are being targeted towards particular objectives and calls for proposals in specific areas are sought on a regular basis.

The first task is to find an appropriate body to which to apply for funds. Major grant opportunities are advertised in the main scientific press. There are several guides to charitable funding bodies which should be found in the local medical library. Major academic institutions provide information from central research support units which publish listings of available grants. Most major hospitals and universities have similar units which publish internal listings of available grants with deadlines and can also give help in completing the application forms.

PATIENT CONSENT FORM

ALCAP TRIAL IN METASTATIC PROSTATE CANCER

Hospital Number:

I ....,

of ....,

agree to take part in a trial of treatment in prostate cancer. I understand that treatment will be randomly allocated to me but that if my doctor or I feel the treatment to be inappropriate, standard treatment will be given.

I understand that if I do not agree to enter this trial, my rights to treatment will not be affected.

I understand that I may withdraw from this trial at any time if I wish, and withdrawal will not affect my rights to treatment and appropriate care.

I have been given a full explanation of the trial, and have received a written explanation.

Signed .... Date ....

CONFIRMATION OF EXPLANATION BY CLINICIAN

I, ..., (position held ....)

confirm that I have given a full explanation of the trial to... and have also given him/her a written explanation.

Signed .... Date ....

WITNESS TO THE SIGNATURE

I, ..., (position held ....)

confirm that a full verbal explanation of the trial has been given to .... I consider that he/she has understood the explanation. He/she has had opportunity to ask questions

Signed .... Date ....

Figure 4.18 Model patient consent form

PATIENT INFORMATION SHEET FOR THE ALCAP TRIAL IN METASTATIC PROSTATIC CARCINOMA.

Your doctor has already explained that you have cancer of the prostate gland and that some cancer cells have spread into your bones. The doctor will also have explained what this means for you.

You will be commencing or have already received the standard therapy for your disease. Some doctors believe that by altering the composition of bone the cancer cells will find it harder to grow and cause damage. This has not been tested in large numbers of patients yet. Finding a medicine that will penetrate bone and stay there without causing any harm is difficult.

There are, however, medicines already available which do get into bone. Such a medicine is called antileukin. It is already used in patients who may have problems due to the spread of their cancer.

You have been invited to take part in a trial in which we want to find out whether by giving antileukin to men like you we can prevent or at least slow down the consequences of the cancer cells in bones. We must compare what happens to patients who take antileukin with patients who do not take the medicine. This will take a few years.

Patients who agree to participate in this trial will be allocated by chance (basically "drawing the treatment out of a hat") to either antileukin or a placebo (a non-active form) in addition to the standard treatment you are getting now. For every patient who participates this means taking four tablets per day every day, for up to three years. Some patients who have taken antileukin have had mild diarrhoea and felt sick and occasionally experienced a mild skin rash, a low white blood cell count or a low calcium level. If this happens to you, your tablets will be reduced or stopped altogether. Your other treatment will be exactly the same whether you enter the trial or not.

You must be aware that by agreeing to take part in this study you may not directly gain any benefit from it. The results will, however, be of value to other patients in the future.

If you do not wish to take part in this trial or if you wish to withdraw at any time you will continue to receive the standard treatment. Your relationship with your doctors will not be affected in any way. If you do agree to take part and you subsequently wish to withdraw from the trial at any time, again you will be free to do so. This will not affect your treatment.

If you agree to take part in the trial your family doctor will be informed.

Figure 4.19 Model patient information sheet.

Sets of forms and guidelines on the grant application process are obtainable from the funding bodies such as the MRC. Research support units may hold these on file which can save a great deal of individual effort. Major bodies tend to use a two stage commissioning process. A short initial application is requested which goes through a first round selection procedure. These applications generally cover 2 - 4 sides of A4 paper and include outline details of the research proposed and the support required. A good example is the NHS R&D funding programme. At this stage the results of the selection process will either be acceptance, a suggestion of referral elsewhere, perhaps to a more suitable programme, or rejection. If rejected, a resumé of the reasons for rejection is usually given and one may be able to challenge the decision if it is felt to be unjust. However, it is more likely that the reasons will be valid and applicants are well advised to accept the criticisms and to modify the application accordingly before re-submission or submission elsewhere. Indeed, it may be very constructive in these circumstances to seek the advice of the grant giving body as to how to modify the proposal; it is sometimes surprising how helpful they can be. This would be particularly true for research commissioned at a local level and one role of the recently appointed regional and trust level research directors is to provide such advice.

If selected to enter the second round, a fuller application will be requested and it is now necessary to provide exact details of the research proposed and the resources required. Though the odds of success shorten at this stage, the degree of scrutiny increases so the production of this second stage proposal can be much more difficult than the first. The major headings of the MRC application forms are shown below. This indicates the level of detail typically required at this stage and for the newcomer it is recommended that advice is sought on this process from an experienced senior colleague. It is imperative that the form is completed to the letter as any anomalies, however small, will detract from the chances of success.

If the planning stages suggested above have been followed, most of the information required will be at hand and will be well constructed. The details which present problems at this stage are generally to do with financial details. Overheads are a particular bug-bear and relate to a levy applied to grants to cover the infrastructure costs of the institution in which work is carried out. The size and scope of overheads varies from place to place and from grant-giving body to grant-giving body. Essentially, it is usual to add a fixed percentage (up to 40 - 50% in some cases) to the total salary bill of the grant concerned. This can be a sizeable amount of money which can give the cost-benefit equation a new perspective! Check carefully about overheads, however, as grantgiving bodies are moving increasingly towards full cost grants which normally include the overhead costs, post, photocopying, office expenses and secretarial help, each of which have to be itemised. European grants pose special problems as regards overheads and expenses as EC contractual arrangements can be extremely complex and it is recommended that experienced help is sought before embarking on such projects.

1. Details of applicants

2. Institution administering grant

3. Title of investigation (116 characters maximum)

4. Type of grant sought

5. Abstract of research (250 words)

6. Start date and duration

7. Summary of support requested broken down by year and category (staff, consumables, equipment etc.)

8. Statement of ethical approval

9. Declaration by applicants of acceptance of MRC standard conditions

10. Signatures of Head of Department and Administering Authority

11. Address

12. History of proposed research
    Title
    Questions concerning previous / concurrent applications

13. Addresses of applicants

14. Addresses of collaborators

ANNEX 1 PROPOSED INVESTIGATION
        Maximum of five A4 sides for Project Grants / Special Project Grants
        Maximum of nine A4 sides for Programme Grants
Title
Purpose
Background
Plan of Investigation
Detailed justification for support required

ANNEX 2
Detailed breakdown of all costs

ANNEX 3
CV of Applicants, proposed research staff / visiting senior scientist

ANNEX 4
Report on previous MRC Grant(s)
A one A4 page report for grants held by applicants over the preceding 5 years

Figure 4.20   Headings of a current MRC Grant application form

1. Details of lead applicant

2. Project details
      Area of R&D Need
      Project title
      Summary (200 words)
      Duration
      Start date
      Overhead (% of costs)
      Total cost

3. Details of joint applicants

4. Details of proposed investigation

      a. Title
      b. Background to the project
      c. Plan of investigation including research methodology proposed
      d. Benefits the proposed investigation will bring to the NHS
      e. Justification of the support required
      f. References

Figure 4.21 Major headings of a current NHS Grant Form

IDENTIFYING COLLABORATORS

Collaborators will generally be drawn from within a circle of colleagues, often based in the same institution. With the complexity of medical problems research teams are often formed from multidisciplinary groupings. When putting together a project it is worth considering whether additional specialist input would be helpful and seeking it out if necessary. Health economics is becoming an essential component of much NHS research and if a project lacks the relevant expertise in this area a grant submission is more likely to fail. Similarly, many Research Council initiatives and the European Union programmes demand partnerships with industrial organisations and across national boundaries. Working with such groups can be invigorating. Sometimes, however, the extra management burden and the conflict of academic and commercial interests can create unexpected frustrations.

A current issue which is worth considering at this stage is the likely involvement in co-authorship of any publications produced by the project. Early agreement on this can avoid problems of grant holders expecting automatic right of inclusion on papers when their actual scientific involvement has been minimal, for example in cases where they have merely enabled access to a particular patient group. The International Committee of

Medical Journal Editors (the Vancouver group) has published guidelines for inclusion as authors which could be useful in setting a yardstick for discussions with potential collaborators. In short, working in the right team with clearly defined individual responsibilities is essential. Collaborators should be chosen with care!

HOW IS A RESEARCH PROPOSAL EVALUATED?

Though the emphasis in this section has been on how to run studies, in time one may be asked to evaluate studies for grant-giving bodies or ethics committees. It is worth considering the mechanism by which this is carried out at an early stage as by understanding the method of appraisal it is more likely that pitfalls in grant proposals can be avoided.

In most cases proposals submitted to grant-giving bodies are peer reviewed by a moderate sized panel of scrutineers. They will evaluate the proposal and usually score it against a relatively tight set of criteria. Once all the grants are scored they are ranked and the available money allocated. In all the cases it is important that the submissions are of high quality and follow the criteria set by the grant-awarding body as generally proposals will be eliminated on a sudden death basis.

Figure 4.22 is based on the kind of checklist that reviewers use when reading grants and gives an indication of how failings would lead to rejections. It is obvious that the scientific or clinical question being addressed should be of significance but this is not the only criterion which is used. The application itself must be of high scientific quality, stating the problems clearly and using published evidence intelligently to support its cause. The proposal must be realistic, especially in terms of being achievable with the resources requested. Where needed, appropriate collaboration must be identified as discussed previously.

EXECUTION

RECRUITING THE SUBJECTS/ FINDING THE SPECIMENS

This is not as easy as it sounds. Researchers rarely have complete control of their subjects even in animal research. Unexpected contingencies frequently crop up and recruitment is always slower than would be predicted theoretically from the study design. With this in mind the elapsed time of projects has a tendency to stretch beyond initial target end points. One often has to rely on colleagues to identify potential patients or samples and diplomacy and constant gentle encouragement are needed in copious amounts. This is especially true if the research is to be carried out on patients or samples presenting through routine clinical channels. Invariably, the one sample that would be ideal for study is the one that has been lost, broken in the centrifuge or has too small a volume to be of use. Attention paid to creating fail-safes and back-ups at this stage will pay off well in the end since without the raw material little else can be achieved.

Grant Item	Criteria	Comments
Title	Does the title make sense and adequately summarise the project?	Though failure is unlikely because of a poor title, a misleading or ambiguous title will not help the case.
Summary	Does the summary adequately encapsulate the research problem? Does it include all the significant information?	Again, though failure is unlikely on a poor summary alone, in the heat of the grant arbitration meeting a poor or confused summary will not help to support the case.
Benefits of research	Is it clearly stated who will benefit from the research and in what way?	Much research and particularly NHS research is goal directed, failing to justify why the research will be of value will weaken the case.
Purpose of research	Is the problem clearly stated?	Ask an experienced colleague unfamiliar with the research topic to check this.
Background	Does the background material adequately summarise the current state of knowledge? Does it indicate where the current project fits into prior research programmes? Does it indicate a logical progression? Does it show a clear understanding of relevant literature in the field?	Ask an experienced colleague unfamiliar with the research topic to check this.
Hypothesis	Is/are there a clearly stated hypothesis/hypo-theses? Does this follow logically from the research problem? If proven will they answer the research question?	Ask an experienced colleague unfamiliar with the research topic to check this.

Figure 4.22   Grant evaluation checklist

Grant Item	Criteria	Comments
Plan of investigation	Is there a steering group/management organisation to control the project? Is the plan clear, unambiguous and feasible? Does it address the hypothesis/hypotheses? Is the experimental model sound? Are all relevant data items to be collected properly identified? Is the experiment ethical and if necessary has ethics approval been obtained? Are adequate methods for randomisation, double/single blinding etc. identified? Are the proposed control and study groups appropriate for the experiment? Have the correct methods been used to ident-ify the sample sizes and power of the study? Are the sample sizes considered: too small (fails on statistical grounds) or too big (fails on ethical grounds because of unnecessary risks to subjects)?	Most of these are check list items but in some cases (ethical permission; statistical calculations) expert advice should be sought.
Justification of support requested	Are the resources identified in the proposal necessary to carry out the research? Do they fall within the remit of the grant? Does the Institution / Research Team have the resources and facilities to undertake the work proposed?	Note some grant bodies exclude certain items, e.g. PCs, capital items
Miscellaneous	Is the research contingent on other factors? Is permission needed to use other facilities, access to patients / materials not under the direct control of the research team?	Any permissions needed should be clearly stated and documentary evidence may be required that they have been obtained.
Past record	Do the researchers have a good past record; papers published? projects completed?	A short CV is usually needed for most applications. In some cases this will be a personal CV for each member of the team. In other cases an Institutional CV may be needed.
Methods of dissemination	Are the methods of dissemination clearly identified? Are they feasible? Is there a mechanism for follow-up and review of the project?	Most grant giving bodies now ask for information as to how the research findings will be published, disseminated and exploited. They also now expect to receive regular progress reports and a final report on the outcome. In the review process 'products', especially peer-reviewed publications of findings, are rated highly and will be expected. Failure to produce these will reflect badly on researchers applying for follow-up grants or new proposals.

Figure 4.22   Grant evaluation checklist (continued)

GAINING INFORMED CONSENT

Obtaining informed consent from subjects is a very important step in study execution and demands tact and understanding. The issue of ethical approval has been discussed above along with the questions of appropriate forms and information sheets (page 158). If the former step has been successfully negotiated the practical recruitment should be made more straightforward. The essential maxim is that the decision of the patient is final and though they may be enthusiastically encouraged to take part such encouragement should not leave them feeling pressured. If this is the case they will invariably withdraw at the first opportunity and valuable early work will be wasted. It is better to have a willing and compliant group of subjects than one which is even marginally recalcitrant.

In some cases it is recommended that informed consent be obtained by someone independent of the study to ensure fair play. Whether this is necessary should have been considered during the planning stage and all the necessary procedures instituted. Certainly it is wise to leave the patients with sufficient time to discuss the matter with relatives in privacy before expecting a decision.

COLLECTING DATA

Though computers are viewed as the modern method of data collection, two traditional tools of the trade deserve mention here: laboratory notebooks and structured data forms. Computers are dealt with later (page 174).

LABORATORY NOTEBOOKS

The appropriate use of laboratory notebooks is an essential discipline. Keeping a notebook as a kind of day-by-day log can save a lot of trouble when reviewing a piece of research or project work. It is all too easy to forget small details which may have an important bearing on the interpretation of results at the analysis stage. For example, changing the composition of a buffer or the type of standard employed in an assay can critically affect results. Although it is easy to think such things can be remembered, when looking back confusion often rules.

Though loose leaf folders are convenient for storing experimental results, there is a major danger of losing the order of pages unless they are individually dated. A hard back notebook with dated pages helps to maintain the chronology of experiments. Sometimes the record of an apparently trivial observation can assume major significance when reviewing a series of experiments.

FORMS

It is good experience to study one of the protocol booklets produced by drug companies for use in clinical trials. Due to the rigorous audit of such trials, particularly by the FDA in the USA, these provide an excellent model for data collection procedures. Companies go to great lengths to ensure that data collection is both complete and predictable. Paying attention to this aspect of the study at an early stage will save much time and effort later. A main feature of such booklets is the use of structured data forms.

The design of a clear and appropriate set of forms will do much to enhance the quality of data collected (though not necessarily its relevance!). Forms also make it easier to identify gaps early on in the study and mitigate against missing data points which could invalidate the whole study by, for example, the failure to meet randomization criteria. They also greatly aid in organising the data once collected for analysis, either for entry into a computer database or for manual transcription and tabulation before analysis. Forms may even contribute at the planning stage of a study: a dummy run on notional data may reveal deficiencies in the dataset or the procedures for its collection and analysis.

Forms should always have adequate space for the date and time and patient identification that is prominently positioned so that it cannot be overlooked One of the most essential factors is positive identification of the origin and method of collection of each piece of data.

ANALYSING DATA

It is difficult to make categorical statements about the data analysis phase. If the study has gone according to plan then the primary methods of analysis will already have been identified at the planning stage. Difficulties arise if datasets are incomplete or the results are unexpected. In this case an imaginative and exploratory approach must be adopted to conduct further analysis in the light of modified hypotheses. Trawling through data in the hope of hitting significant 'P' values is strongly discouraged. Splitting the datasets into subgroups to achieve similar goals is an equally flawed activity especially since the lower numbers reduce the power of any outcome measure. Attempting sub-group analysis should dictate the need for larger rather than smaller numbers of subjects.

Data should always be plotted before statistical analysis (Chapter 1). Large differences between groups will stand out immediately, as will association between different variables if the data is plotted appropriately. The usual problem is of being able *to see the wood for the trees* especially if the datasets are large. Plotting a few graphs sometimes quickly alerts the researcher to the major findings and allows the analysis to be appropriately orientated.

Often at this stage the requirement for further or deeper analysis is generated and one must be prepared to return to the primary data, checking for accuracy and reconsidering assumptions and conclusions. Though highlighted here as a sequential task, data analysis is intimately bound into the reporting process.

REPORTING

"A man is a teller of tales, he lives surrounded by his stories and the stories of others, he sees everything that happens to him through them; and he tries to live his life as if he were recounting it."

Jean-Paul Sartre

Reporting scientific work can be very exacting. To put over a complex argument with clarity and brevity calls for good communication skills. It can also be great fun and provide immense satisfaction, particularly if presented to an interested audience in an exotic location! However the scrutiny of peers can also be particularly cruel, exposing weaknesses in argument and design and at times proving totally demoralising. For the beginner a useful approach is to present verbally first to local colleagues, then to develop the material for a poster before finally completing the finished paper for publication. Going through these stages allows the work to be gradually polished and reshaped. The criticisms and results of discussion can be incorporated at each reworking, and it is surprising how much a tale improves on each retelling.

WRITING AN ABSTRACT

An abstract may well be the first form of publication of data from a research trial as submitting material to conferences is often an initial way of seeking public exposure. The presentation will usually be as a poster but it may, under some circumstances, be a verbal presentation. A good abstract should describe the research project adequately, include an outline of the data obtained and present clear conclusions. For most conferences, abstracts are scrutinised by a scientific committee who will select appropriate work for either oral or poster presentation. It is important, therefore, that the abstract is attractively and clearly presented, so that under scrutiny it will stand up to the competition.

Abstracts are usually written within a strict word limit or, alternatively, presented in camera-ready form within a limited space. Most conferences reject abstracts which do not contain hard data and are unlikely to accept abstracts which include phrases such as "data will be presented and discussed" without having hard numbers to back up any assertions which are made.

For camera-ready abstracts it is sometimes convenient to include tables of data but it is probably best to avoid graphs since abstracts are often photo-reduced and such graphs appear very small on the printed page. Writing a structured abstract is sometimes helpful, as headings can allow information to be compressed into a small space (see page 137).

PRODUCING A POSTER

Most scientific presentations at conferences are now made in poster format. The main reasons for creating a poster are, firstly to present the work to peers and, secondly to engage in discussions with individuals who may have a common interest and who are likely to provide helpful criticism of the methods and results. This can be useful in the production of the finished paper, as the arguments can be tested on peers in a constructive manner. A poster presentation may well generate new ideas for further research projects or even create collaborative research groupings.

It is important to gain experience in poster production. There is no correct way to create a poster and, indeed, the most appropriate format will depend upon the type of material being presented. There are, however, many mistakes which can be made and the following guidelines will be helpful.

Clear and informative headings are essential. The tendency is for delegates at conferences to browse through the poster section, stopping at posters which catch their eye. Therefore a clear, attractive layout and eye catching informative headings can do much to attract attention. As a guide, the general lettering on a poster should be readable at a distance of 1 metre (18 pt) and headings (36 pt or 24 pt) should be scaled appropriately larger. On the whole, it is better to rely on visual aids such as graphs and tables than on large amounts of detailed text.

TITLE SIZE
TEXT SIZE FOR A SUBTITLE
Text size suitable for main paragraphs of a poster presented at a Scientific Meeting

---

A poster should present information in an attractive and easily read form, saving detailed information for an appendix. For example, extensive details of methods are best avoided unless they are pertinent to the main scientific argument.

Introduction	Brief outline of objectives of research project plus major aims
Methods	Short description of general method and approach.
Results	Clear exposition of results, in tables or, preferably, figures.
Discussion	Brief section on major points of interest.
Conclusions	Best set out as a list of bullet points.

Figure 4.23 Major headings for a poster

The physical appearance of a poster can vary from hand-drawn and hand-written material through computer-generated material mounted on backing sheets to elaborately printed, large scale colour output. One sometimes wonders if the costs of such productions can be justified when the material may well be displayed for only an hour or two and looked at in any detail by perhaps less than one hundred individuals. The most valuable part of the exercise, however, is likely to be the thought that goes into designing and creating the poster, selecting the information to present, and structuring it in a way that can be rapidly and easily assimilated. This process can be an important step on the way towards producing a final, definitive publication of research findings.

GIVING AN ORAL PRESENTATION

The next step beyond the poster presentation of scientific material is oral presentation. The format is usually a fifteen minute slot in a rolling scientific programme, perhaps twelve minutes presentation and three minutes questioning. The skill in such a situation is to summarise a large amount of data in a short time whilst maintaining clarity and coherence. With appropriate structuring and attention to the development of the argument, a great deal of information can be presented within the twelve minute period, particularly if audio-visual materials are well designed and developed.

The general structure of such a presentation would be to outline the background and objectives of the research project, to give some background data, to create a context to the work, to indicate the main methodology and present a summary of the results, drawing conclusions appropriately from the data so presented. It is important to pitch the presentation at the correct level for the intended audience, that is, to neither under-estimate nor overestimate their background knowledge of the subject, and not to pursue the argument at too superficial or too sophisticated a level.

An essential preparatory step is to give the talk on several occasions to local peers and colleagues before presentation at any public event. This rehearsal and the constructive criticism received from colleagues will do much to improve not only the content but also the style of presentation. By the time the final presentation is made one should be so comfortable with the material as to be able to give the presentation with very little stress or nervousness. Fielding any questions will be a good deal easier, as most of the obvious ones will already have been asked by colleagues. It may be useful to offer the chairperson of the session a question one would like to receive. Chairpersons will often be quite relieved to be given such a question since, if the interest of the audience has not been excited, it will fall to them to open and maintain some discussion. Indeed, many experienced chairpersons will ask presenters what question they would like to be asked in order to give them an easier opening to the question session.

The use of visual aids is a vexed question and competence with projectors both slide and overhead varieties is under-rated and sadly lacking in many scientists. McLuhan may have been scientifically incorrect in his assertion that 'the medium is the massage' but poor presentation greatly devalues a scientific message and does little to enhance the presenters image and standing amongst peers. Attending a course on presentation skills is highly recommended and will have many benefits in related areas such as teaching. It is far better to get over the pain of criticism of presentation styles in the relative anonymity of a seminar room or video studio than in a major plenary session at a national or international conference.

On the day of a presentation it is advisable to arrive early at the venue to check the room and the audio-visual systems in advance. There is little consistency in the layout of control mechanisms and under the stress of the event it is easy to become confused by an array of control buttons on a badly lit lectern. Familiarity with microphones also helps and a sound check may seem like overkill but is worth it if the 15 minutes of exposure is to be fully exploited. When giving a talk it is a disaster if the audio-visual system fails. Thorough rehearsal can help one to be prepared for this eventuality since, if one is familiar with the material, it should be possible to *ad lib* even without the slides. Recourse to a pen and overhead projector, or even chalk and blackboard, can be very effective and impressive. The actual content and quality of slides is discussed in the section below.

WRITING A PROJECT REPORT

This will often be the first exposure to writing up a piece of scientific work. Scientists may have been gained experience at degree level but it is more likely that a clinician's first experience of a report of this type will be for a higher degree such as MRCPath. The standard format will be to write up the work in standard sections of:

- Introduction
- Methods and materials
- Results
- Discussion
- Conclusions
- References

Before starting it is important to read the instructions provided by the examining body very carefully, particularly for the number of words required and the style used for references. Sometimes a short abstract is required.

If the project is to be examined then one aim is to produce a report which indicates a scientific approach to a problem and a level of general competence in scientific writing. The value of the findings of the project is less important. Indeed, at this level many projects will have produced inconclusive or negative results and thus marks depend more on approach and style than on conclusions. Attention to detail is essential. The past tense should be used throughout and spelling, punctuation and references should be meticulously checked.

The introduction may take the form of a short literature review or a long essay. As with a research grant application, a logical argument should be presented leading up to the development of the hypothesis to be tested and an explanation of the relevance of the practical work undertaken. All assertions should be backed up with a reference to the relevant literature and vague statements of scientific truths are best avoided. Obtaining second hand arguments from review articles can be dangerous and it is always better to read and refer to the original papers.

Compared with a paper, the materials and methods section should contain much more detailed information about the procedures used. Indeed, many projects do not get much beyond a methodological study and hence a detailed account of the stages of development of an assay and the associated validation procedures may be needed.

The results section should give a clear account of the results obtained including any negative ones if relevant, and should include the statistical information. Any commentary should be reserved for the discussion. A fairly direct, factual style is to be encouraged here.

In the discussion section the results are placed in context and assessed in relation to the hypothesis under test and the existing information on the subject. Negative results should be covered as well as positive ones since these can indicate how much understanding the candidate has of the subject matter. It is as well to end with a short conclusion and to include in this suggestions about further experiments that could be pursued on the basis of the new data obtained.

WRITING A THESIS

Writing a thesis is the next step up from a project report but is several orders of magnitude more difficult. It will embody a much larger body of work and the process will be much more difficult to control. The process will also extend over a much longer period and maintaining consistency presents extra problems.

The format is much the same as that for a project report but the level of detail will be much greater. The introduction will be expected to be a definitive literature review of the subject area and to contain a very complete exposition of the background to the subject of the research project.

The exact layout will depend on the type of material to be included. In some cases a series of experiments may be presented as a set of chapters sandwiched between a general introduction and a final discussion chapter.

As with a project report, it is important before starting work to consult the regulations of the examining institution as these vary a good deal. Some have strict rules for layout and word limits and breaching the rules will result in the need for a painful rewrite or even outright failure. As many examiners now require revisions and corrections to be completed before final acceptance, soft-binding may be needed at the point of initial submission with hard binding following successful examination.

In addition to its scientific value, a thesis is a test of the scholarship of the author. As a consequence the attention paid by the examiners to spelling, punctuation, accuracy of references and scientific conventions, such as abbreviations used for units, is high. Theses do not fail on the basis of spelling alone but sloppy presentation will not impress examiners and will be punished by the need for extensive revisions. It is better to get this right at the beginning than to have to revisit a piece of work many times to correct trivial errors.

It is advisable to find a sympathetic and experienced supervisor and to have work reviewed progressively during the period of the research project. PhD students are allocated a supervisor who is *required* to review work periodically. Students for some post-graduate degrees such as MDs do not normally have official supervisors but are strongly advised to find a "mentor" who can fulfill this role. Leaving the writing up to the end of a period of research is not a good practice. Methods can be written up immediately they are used and the discipline of doing this can help reveal flaws before it is too late. Similarly, maintaining an ongoing literature review to keep up with the field of work reduces the pressure when completing the project against time limits.

WRITING A PAPER

Writing a full paper is a difficult task, though if the data has already been through the cycle of an abstract, poster or oral presentation much of the hard work will already have been carried out. People have different and unique approaches to this problem and papers often cycle through several drafts before reaching a stage where the manuscript is ready to be presented to a journal. Writing an initial structured abstract (see above) is always a good way to get ideas focused especially if multiple authors are involved.

The classic style of abstract, introduction, methods, results, discussion and references is that required by most journals.

The first task is usually to summarise the data for the results section, since this is the principal output of the data analysis phase of the research project. The tables and graphs which are felt to be essential to the argument should be prepared at an early stage and then the text built around them. Deciding whether data should be in tables or in the narrative can be quite tricky. Some journals limit the number of tables and figures that can be included and this may force the issue of what goes where. It may help in deciding which findings are essential to include in a table by considering how one might summarise the results as slides in a talk. If this could be achieved by including one or two tables from the paper, then the correct balance will have been achieved.

The method section is generally the next area to complete, largely because it should be a relatively simple process to explain what was done and how the research was conducted. Appropriate attention to detail is needed. In the main, existing methods do not need to be described in detail but should be clearly referenced. Where substantial modifications have been introduced however these should be covered to the level where another worker could repeat the work from the description provided. If methodological issues form a significant component of the research then these should be highlighted and will probably deserve mention in the introduction and discussion.

The current emphasis on evidence-based medicine is influencing the style of presentation of scientific data. In order that information can be included in systematic reviews and meta-analyses there is a growing requirement to include background information which previously might have been thought superfluous. In part this information is needed to convince readers of the veracity of the work undertaken but in part is also needed such that data can be combined across papers. In the particular case of diagnostic test evaluation a recent review in JAMA has delineated seven key methodological standards by which papers in this area can be judged (Reid *et al*, 1995). The review concluded that only a minority of publications met the standards and that there was room for much improvement in reporting practice. It can be expected that similar standards will soon be established in relation to other areas of study and also that these standards will be applied rigorously by the editors and referees of scientific journals. Note that all the standards listed in Figure 4.24 have been highlighted in earlier sections on test evaluation and experimental design.

1. Specify spectrum of patients studied (ages, genders, diseases etc)

2. Report test indices (reference ranges) for subgroups studied

3. Avoid workup bias (randomise and blind patient selection)

4. Avoid review bias (blind assessment)

5. Provide numerical precision for test indices

6. Report on frequency and handling of outliers

7. Specify test reproducibility (accuracy and imprecision)

From: Heaton R, Smith R.
Signing up for authorship. *Lancet* 1996; **347:** 780

Figure 4.24   Seven key methodological standards for reporting diagnostic test research

The introduction and discussion will follow and may need simultaneous revision in order to give the paper the correct shape. Clearly, if the research project has gone through the planning stages indicated above, the introduction will largely follow from the background research conducted at the beginning. Introductions to papers are shorter than thesis introductions, however, and tend to place work in context rather than present a detailed review.

Having written the bulk of the paper, the final jobs will be the production of an adequate abstract and checking the accuracy of references. Several methods are used for references though most journals now subscribe to the Vancouver style.

It is essential to follow to the letter the publisher's guidelines for the journal to which the paper is to be submitted, detail such as the format of units (SI or non-SI) being of particular importance. Journals carry instructions to authors routinely, sometimes in every issue and sometimes only once a year. An example is the Annals of Clinical Biochemistry where they are included on each inside back cover. For another complete set see any January issue of Clinical Chemistry which has a detailed and well-referenced set of instructions including advice on statistical methods. Failure to follow such instructions is likely to lead to almost immediate rejection. Journals have no shortage of submitted material and, given the work involved in the refereeing and editing process, many journals will not take the trouble to consider badly presented work which is at variance with their house style. However, an exception is often made when the work comes from a country where the national language is not English.

RESPONDING TO THE REFEREES' REPORTS

Unless a paper is exceptional the response to a submitted paper will be a list of referees' criticisms of the work presented. This should not be unexpected as it is the job of the referees to critically review the submitted material and they are unlikely to agree with everything anyone submits. It is not uncommon to feel that they have entirely missed the point, even to the extent of suspecting that they have not read the paper in detail. This is rarely the case and if they have missed the point then there is likely to be a flaw in the argument or in the way it has been presented. Disagreements between referees do occur and in these circumstances an editor will often seek another opinion so that the comments returned will represent a consensus view.

The best approach is to accept the response in as constructive a light as possible and to consider modifications to the paper which will address the issues raised. Usually the criticisms can be accommodated in this way and a revised version of the paper will be accepted with little or no further modification.

Where there is serious disagreement, entering into a dialogue with the editor is worthwhile. It will often then be necessary to present a point by point rebuttal of the criticisms, possibly presenting new or independent supporting evidence. In our experience entering a constructive debate on these lines can be extremely rewarding both for the enjoyment of the cut and thrust of scientific debate and for the fact that the focus and sharpness of the paper invariably improves in the process.

An interesting development made possible by the rapid expansion of the internet are several experiments of on-line peer review. The Medical Journal of Australia allows papers and expert refereed comments to be viewed on the World Wide Web and readers can submit comments which are sent to authors before final editing of the printed publication. Clinical Endocrinology now allows papers to be viewed on-line before publication and similarly invites readers' comments. In addition it prints the correspondence generated within the same issue as the main paper thereby overcoming a problem inherent in scientific publishing that relevant criticisms and comments may be overlooked as they appear in different issues of the journal.

SUBMITTING PUBLISHED WORKS FOR HIGHER DEGREES
Some institutions, universities and Royal Colleges allow higher degrees to be gained by the submission of published works. In the past this has sometimes been seen as a soft option. With increasing pressure to justify research ratings, which are partly measured on quality of graduate output, the criteria have become more stringent. Indeed, amassing sufficient material to succeed by this route is not a trivial task when one considers the amount of work which is required to produce a single worthwhile paper. The usual process is to approach the institution with a request to submit for a degree in this way. Sometimes they will conduct an initial assessment of a simple list of publications to see whether there is a *prima facie* case to proceed further. If this is successful then the applicant is expected to present a copy of the papers to be considered accompanied by a commentary on the work they contain. This is intended to explain the significance of the work and, if possible, demonstrate any themes which bind them together into a logical

corpus of work of academic merit. It is usually also necessary to provide supporting evidence that the bulk of the work presented represents the personal contribution of the applicant and to clarify the contributions made by others. With the trend towards multi-authored papers containing work generated by multidisciplinary groups it can sometimes be hard to clearly identify sources for the intellectual content of many papers. This is another reason why this method of examination is used less and less.

VIVA VOCE

It is difficult to consider production of reports and theses for examinations without also touching on viva voce examinations. This is the occasion when examiners have a chance to question the applicant directly about the content of their work. Any deficiencies in the work and its presentation will be highlighted in the discussion and, unless meticulous attention has been paid to detail, even minor spelling and punctuation errors can cause grief. The main purpose of the *viva voce* should be to have a lively debate about the scientific merits of the work and to spoil this through negligent presentation is unforgivable. Proof reading is difficult and it pays to ask for help from a supervisor, colleague or friend, as identifying even glaring errors in material with which one is very familiar can be extremely difficult.

This section has attempted to cover the difficult areas of experimental design and execution. The diversity of scientific problems and the numerous approaches available for study makes it impossible to provide prescriptive rules for success. Science is a creative process and innovation on the part of scientists and researchers is to be strongly encouraged. We hope however that we will have provided some way-markers in this section which will help the novice to chart an initial course into the world of scientific discovery. For the more experienced we hope that our comments will resonate with previous experience and perhaps stimulate re-assessment of approaches and re-invigorate curiosity.

COMPUTERS - ESSENTIAL TOOLS OF THE TRADE

It is unlikely that the modern clinical scientist will survive without at least rudimentary information technology (IT) skills. Though it is possible to conduct studies without using computers for planning, data storage, analysis or reporting it is less and less likely that this will be the case. Therefore, the developing scientist should seek to become competent in computer use. How competent is a vexed question. Like all tools, computers need to be used correctly to produce optimal results. They can be extremely distracting. The ease with which the formats of documents, diagrams and databases can be revised may dissipate energy which should be focused on content rather than appearance. The most efficient word processor is probably a combination of a dictaphone, a secretary skilled in the use of a personal computer (PC) and a red pencil, an approach frequently taken with the manuscript of this book! However, access to such secretarial facilities is nowadays limited and PC self-sufficiency is more often the rule. A list of IT skills which might be expected of a scientist is given in Figures 4.25 and 4.26. They are divided into those which one could consider essential and those which would be desirable extras.

Essential skills	Ability level
Word-processing	Basic text formatting Creation of tables Insertion and editing of references (endnotes)
Database use	Data entry Report generation Data selection and manipulation
Spreadsheet use	Data entry Rudimentary calculation using formulae
Statistics	Data entry Data analysis
Graphics and drawing	Production of graphs and diagrams for publication Production of slides

Figure 4.25   Essential IT skills for a scientist

Desirable skills	Ability level
Word-processing	Creation of forms Creation of questionnaires
Database use	Creation of database specifications Import / export of data to other packages, e.g. spreadsheets, word-processors, graphics
Literature searching	Use of Medline - on-line or via CD-ROM Storage of references on disk files
Bibliographic database use	Importation of references to personal database Generation of bibliographies

Figure 4.26   Desirable IT skills for a scientist

WORD PROCESSORS

Most people now have access to a word processor and there are dozens from which to choose. The leading packages are Microsoft Word and WordPerfect and the choice is a matter of personal preference. There is little difference between the features available in any particular package and most of the more powerful functions are rarely used.

Important features to consider when choosing or learning how to use a package include techniques available for constructing and manipulating tables and the availability of special fonts including Greek and scientific characters. Struggling to format tables with tabs will drive many people to their wits end and learning to use the table formatting tools of a package like Word can save hours of work.

Other features which are worth learning, especially when preparing a thesis, are the use of stylesheets and outlines. These can help greatly with consistency of layout and in reorganising sections of material within a large document. As an aside, the preparation of this book has relied heavily on these features, especially in merging material from the two co-authors.

DATABASES

Most users are familiar with word processors and adapt easily to the tabular nature of spreadsheets, but fail to appreciate that databases offer far more powerful and flexible functions for data storage and analysis.

Whereas word-processed documents and spreadsheets have fixed layouts, databases adopt an approach similar to a card index. Each item is held in a separate record and these records may be selected or reordered at will. This means that subsets of the data can be extracted for analysis without the need for extensive editing. Such functions as counting the number of male or female subjects can be easily conducted with these systems and by using more complex logical searches quite sophisticated analyses can be carried out without any need to re-enter or edit the primary data. Furthermore, the ability of leading packages such as Microsoft Access, Paradox, DataEase and FoxPro to export selected data to spreadsheets or statistical packages means that by combining such packages sophisticated analyses can be conducted with the minimum of effort. Another advantage of the use of databases is that data checking functions can be applied at the time of data entry, ensuring that data is of the correct form and within acceptable credibility limits. Exploitation of this function can help avoid errors, especially in large datasets.

Databases are surprisingly easy to use and it is well worth the effort of learning the rudiments. Though most users will not become highly skilled in database use, in most departments and hospitals help will be available if complex applications are needed for data entry programmes.

REFERENCE DATABASES

In addition to the standard flexible databases such as Microsoft Access or Paradox, a number of other specialist databases are available to help the researcher. Amongst these one would include the reference-handling databases capable of storing references downloaded from Medline or entered by hand to produce a completely personalised information base. Two good examples of these are Reference Manager and Endnote, both freely available and running from both Windows and Macintosh PCs. In addition to their ability to act like an electronic card index, they can also be used at the reporting stage to automatically generate bibliographies for manuscripts, since data can be entered into them electronically from data downloaded from systems such as Medline and CD-ROM reference databases. Thus, much of the laborious typing can be reduced and errors minimised. An extensive review outline on the subject written by one of us is available in the British Medical Journal (Jones, 1993).

SPREADSHEETS

Spreadsheets are essentially computerised tables which include built-in calculation functions. They were initially developed for use by accountants and they have been expanded to include many powerful functions for data analysis such as sorting and some statistical features. Leading examples include the Microsoft Excel package and Lotus 123. They are particularly suitable for carrying out large numbers of repetitive calculations and for the initial stages of data compilation and transformation. They suffer from limitations when applied to large scale data storage and retrieval and are best used for data analysis in conjunction with a database.

STATISTICAL PACKAGES

A large number of statistics packages are available ranging from the very simple to the highly sophisticated PC version of professional systems such as SPSS and SAS. Which package is best will depend upon the problem being addressed, the sophistication of the user and the budget. All the tests described in this book can be found in one or other package but few will contain all of them. For general use we recommend Analyse-IT (Smart Software), a package which is available for use with Microsoft Excel. As it is linked with this popular spreadsheet, it allows data to be handled in an integrated manner with a database such as Access. The package is easy to use. It includes all the tests discussed in previous sections and is available in demo form from the Internet (http://www.smart-software.com) together with many of the datasets used in the examples in this book.

GRAPHICS DRAWING TOOLS

The proper application of the specialist tools provided in graphics package can also be of great benefit. These packages divide into two main groups, those used for the creation of graphs and those used for the production of diagrams. Although many packages are available which will create business graphics, few are capable of generating the sophisticated graphs which may be required for the publication of scientific research. Among those that can produce such graphs are FigP available from Biosoft, and Origin by MicroCal available from Aston Scientific Ltd. More limited graphics capabilities exist in Microsoft Excel but for many purposes these may be perfectly adequate.

One advantage of the business packages is their ability to create presentation slides which can be converted to 35mm format directly from disk. This can greatly help in the preparation of presentations and lectures. If used in conjunction with other Windows or Macintosh-based graphic tools, very powerful visual aids can be produced without undue effort.

For drawings, packages such as Visio, CorelDraw or Micrografix Designer can be used to produce line drawings or other illustrations. However, the time required to learn to use these effectively can be a major disincentive to their use. As with all computer systems the more complex the capability the more complex the package so ease of use must be weighed against sophistication when choosing such packages.

DATA DISPLAY

The major problem with graphics packages is that they are almost too easy to use and poorly designed figures and slides can be mass-produced with ease. To be effective it is necessary to apply rigorously some simple rules which are discussed below. These apply to all graphics but are especially important for slides.

TABLES

The maxim is to keep tables as simple as possible in order to help readers assimilate the information presented. There are no hard and fast rules but by browsing through published papers one soon begins to appreciate the difference between tables which are overloaded with numbers from those that successfully summarise important data. Of course it is sometimes necessary to present complex tables but it is always as well to ask whether less complex layouts would be more effective.

Many methods are used to indicate statistical probabilities which may be associated with data in tables, the exact method used being determined by the house style of the journal. Including such information for the sake of it is unnecessary and including it in the text may be a better option if it detracts from the tabular display. Confidence intervals, which can be indicated in brackets, should be used instead of probability values whenever possible. Each table should have an associated legend describing the content and sometimes drawing attention to the significance of information within it.

GRAPHS

Graphs should be kept simple. Clarity is much more important than a high degree of accuracy. Graphs in papers are illustrations and are too small to use to back-extract data for further analysis. Therefore, one should use bold symbols and lines of sufficient boldness to be well reproduced. In most cases only black and white material is published so effort should not be wasted on complex colour schemes. Similarly, 3D effects should be avoided unless they are necessary to display the information fully as such effects rarely add to a scientific argument. The axes should be clearly labelled with the names of the variables represented together with the relevant units of measurement. The orientation of the axis labels is a matter of personal preference and convenience in slides but is usually a matter of house style in publications. Bear in mind that when graphs are photo-reduced axis labels containing many decimal places can become very small, sometimes to the point of illegibility. Using scientific notation or converting the units to a more manageable form, e.g. g/L to mg/L, can sometimes help.

It is worth producing all graphs at full A4 size if using computer graphics packages and submitting top copy, high quality laser output directly to journals. Printers accept these readily and are able to use them directly. In the past journals required glossy black and white prints but this is not necessary now. Having produced full size graphs it is advisable to photo-reduce them to the size they will be in the journal to check that they are still clear and that the lettering is of the correct size. The percentage reduction in letter size can be quite surprising so it is necessary select large fonts for the original copy.

For graphs a descriptive legend is usually required detailing what the graph illustrates and explaining the significance of any symbols used. Where regression lines or lines of identity are included these are usually mentioned in the legend. Whether the equation for a fitted line is included here, on the graph or in the text will depend on the house style of the journal.

PREPARATION OF ARTWORK FOR SLIDES

One should not be frightened by the term *'artwork'*. Whatever is prepared to be photographed is referred to as *artwork*, however simple it is.

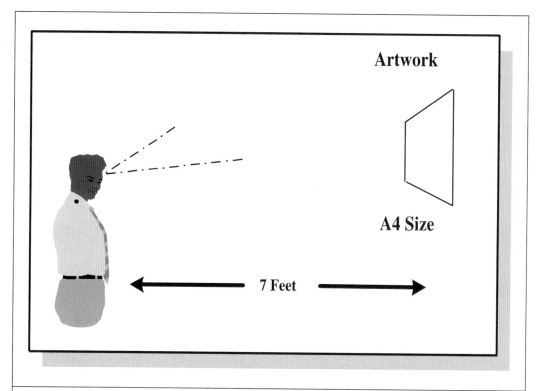

To assess whether artwork for posters or slides will be of the correct size it is best to view it from a distance before committing it for photography. If it is unreadable in these conditions then it will not be legible when projected or mounted as a poster.

Figure 4.27   Assessing artwork

It is extremely common to see bad slides used for lectures and oral presentations. Often it is not for want of effort or skills, and it is hardly ever the fault of the photographer.

The mains faults are:

The slide contains far too much information for the viewer to read

The lettering is too small to read

The colours used do not project well due to lack of colour contrast or saturation.

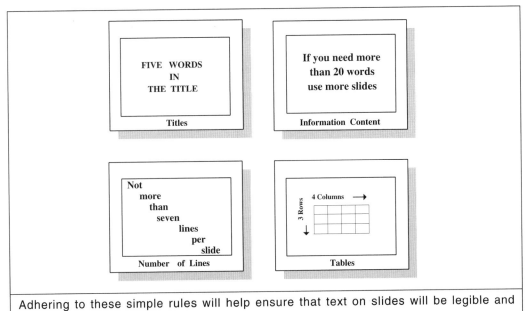

Figure 4.28   Essential rules in creating legible slides

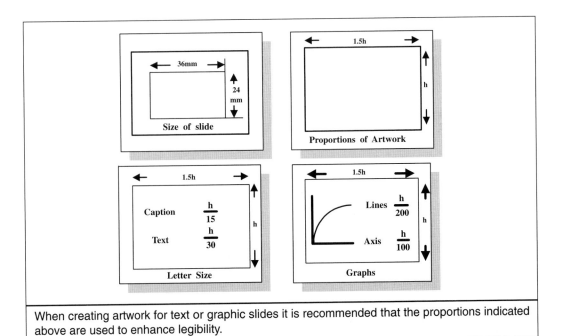

Figure 4.29   Getting the proportions right on artwork for slides

It is rarely possible to make successful slides by copying written or printed material directly from books or papers. The information density is usually far too high. If this is to be attempted consider carefully how the material will look from the back of the room when it is projected.

The same rules apply to computer-generated slides as for ones made from printed graphics. In this case it is additionally important to take care to avoid inappropriate colour combinations. What looks attractive and clear on the screen at a distance of 12 inches can look hopeless when projected on to a large screen. Purples, light blues and reds project very badly unless set against contrasting backgrounds. The physiological constraints of human colour vision make focusing on narrow red lines difficult. Using highly contrasting colours, e.g. white or yellow on a dense blue background, is effective for both text and graphics. Relief from any monotony can be brought by using the occasional cartoon or photograph. The same rules also apply whether the slides are created as 35 mm transparencies or projected directly from a computer through an overhead liquid crystal display (LCD) tablet or video projector.

Since most people now have access to similar computer graphics packages the novelty of fancy backgrounds has worn off, and what might appear attractive to the beginner can seem very hackneyed to the mass of those attending professional conferences who are usually keen to cut through the superficialities to the core scientific content of any talk or presentation.

Above all, keep it simple - do not believe that *'the medium is the massage'* (McLuhan, 1960).

The only way to really learn about computers is to use them. They are not systems which can be learned by rote. One needs to take an exploratory approach and try out different means to reach the desired goal. We have tried to indicate above the potential of some of the specialist tools available from the suppliers listed below. Selecting the correct tool and using it skilfully is the secret of success. Computers are logical beasts. If one approaches them logically then it is possible to avoid the common frustrations.

FURTHER READING

Akawaza K, Odaka T, Sakamoto M, *et al.* A random allocation system with the minimisation method for multi-institutional trials. *J Med Syst* 1991; **15**: 311-9

BMA Ethics, Science and Information Division. *Medical Ethics Today: Its Practice and Philosophy.* London: BMA Publishing Group, 1993

Cochrane A L. *Effectiveness and Efficiency: Random Reflections on Health Services.* London: Nuffield Provincial Hospitals Trust, 1971

Cochrane A L. The history of the measurement of ill health. *Int J Epidemiol* 1972; **1**: 89-92

Crombie, I K, Davies, T O. Towards good audit. *Br J Hosp Med* 1992; **48**: 182-5

Culyer A J, Meads A. The United Kingdom: effective, efficient, equitable? *J Health Polit Policy Law* 1992; **17**: 667-88

Fitzherbert L, Forrester S, Grau J (eds) *A Guide to the Major Trusts.* London: Directory of Social Change,1995

Gill T M, Feinstein. A critical appraisal of the quality of life measurements. *JAMA* 1994; **272**: 619-26

Haynes M E. *Project Management: from Idea to Implementation.* London: Kogan Page, 1989 Kirkwood B R. *Essentials of Medical Statistics.* London: Blackwell Scientific Publications, 1988

Helsinki Declaration 1975 (as revised 1983) in BMA Ethics, Science and Information Division. *Medical Ethics Today: Its Practice and Philosophy.* London: BMA Publishing Group, 1993: Appendix 3

International Committee of Medical Journal Editors. Uniform requirements for manuscripts submitted to biomedical journals. *N Engl J Med* 1991; **324**: 424-28; *Ann Clin Biochem* 1991; **28**: 536-7

Jones R G. Personal computer software for handling CD-ROM and mainframe sources for scientific and medical papers. *BMJ* 1993; **307**: 180-4

Kirkwood B R. *Essentials of Medical Statistics.* London: Blackwell Scientific Publications, 1988

McLuhan M, Fiore, Q. *The Medium is the Massage.* London: Penguin Books, 1967

Pocock S J. *Clinical Trials: a Practical Approach.* Chichester: Wiley and Sons Ltd, 1983

Reid M C, Lachs M S, Feinstein A R. Use of methodological standards in diagnostic test research. *JAMA* 1995; **274**: 645-51

Schulz K F, Chalmers I, Hayes R J, Altman D G. Empirical evidence of bias: dimensions of methodological quality associated with estimates of treatment effects in controlled trials. *JAMA* 1995; **273**: 408-12

Schulz K F, Grimes D A, Altman D G, Hayes R J. Blinding and exclusions after randomised controlled trials: survey of published parallel-group trials in obstetrics and gynaecology. *Br Med J* 1996; **312**: 742-4

Standards of Reporting Trials Group. A proposal for structured reporting of randomised controlled trials. Empirical evidence of bias: dimensions of methodological quality associated with estimates of treatment effects in controlled trials. *JAMA* 1994; **272**: 1926-31

Wasson J H, Reda D J, Bruskewitz R C, Elinson J, Keller A M, Henderson W G. The Veterans Affairs Cooperative Study Group on Transurethral Resection of the Prostate. A comparison of transurethral surgery with watchful waiting for moderate symptoms of benign prostatic hyperplasia. *N Engl J Med* 1995; **332**: 75-9

Williams L (ed). *The Grants Register* (1995-1997), 14th Edition. London: Macmillan Press Ltd, 1994

ARCHIBALD LEMAN COCHRANE

Born Galashiels 12 January 1909. Died Cardiff 18 June 1988.

Archie Cochrane graduated in medicine from UCH in 1938 after spending a year as a medical student with the International Brigade during the Spanish civil war. For four years during the second world war he was a prisoner of war, treating prisoners of many nationalities who had tuberculosis; he became an MBE for this work. After the war he took a DPH and then studied the epidemiology of tuberculosis in America for a year. He then joined the MRC Pneumoconiosis Research Unit at Llandough Hospital near Cardiff where he made his reputation as an epidemiologist, achieving outstanding success in obtaining the co-operation of the population of the Rhondda Fach in South Wales in his research. His earliest studies were on pneumoconiosis. He was acutely aware of the problem of observer error, particularly in the interpretation of radiographs, and helped to devise a series of standard chest films for pneumoconiosis.

In 1960 he was appointed to the David Davies Chair of Chest Diseases and Tuberculosis in the Welsh National School of Medicine. He became a CBE in 1968 for services to medicine. In 1969 he retired from teaching to devote all his time to research as full-time Director of the MRC Epidemiology Research Unit in Cardiff. In 1971 his seminal book *Effectiveness and Efficiency: Random Reflections on Health Services* was published by the Nuffield Provincial Hospitals Trust. In it he wrote that a paper in the BMJ about the value of streptomycin in the treatment of pulmonary tuberculosis "...enabled Bradford Hill to introduce to the medical world the techniques of the randomised controlled trial which added the experimental approach to medical research. Its importance cannot be exaggerated. It opened up a new world of evaluation and control which will, I think, be the key to a rational health service. Freud in his *Zukunft einer Illusion* put his hopes on the gentle voice of intelligence producing order out of another more general chaos. I believe the randomised controlled trial, suitably applied, may have a similar effect in producing an effective, efficient health service." He devoted much of the rest of his life to promoting the virtues of the randomised controlled trial.

The Cochrane Collaboration continues Cochrane's crusade for evidence-based medicine. In 1995 the Department of Health launched the UK Cochrane Database of Systematic Reviews in Oxford to collate evidence-based medical research into an electronic journal. In 1996 this was complemented by the York Database of Abstracts of Reviews of Effectiveness, the Cochrane Controlled Trials Register and the Cochrane Review Methodology Database to form the electronic Cochrane Library.

Archie Cochrane was a small, wiry man with a wicked sense of humour who enjoyed reminiscing about his experiences in the Spanish civil war. He suffered from acute inter-mittent porphyria and had occasional devastating migraines which he explained were an indication of high intelligence. He was one of the first to provide a 'self-written' obituary for the *BMJ*. He ended it by saying that his subject had been "without the consolation of a wife, a religious belief, or a merit award - but he didn't do too badly".

SUPPLIERS OF SCIENTIFIC SOFTWARE

Aston Scientific Ltd
Silverdales House
111 Wendover Road
Stoke Mandeville
Bucks HP22 5TD
UK
Tel: +44 (0)1296 614144
Fax: +44 (0)1296 614228
Email: Origin@astonsci.nildram.co.uk
Web Site: http://www.astonsci.co.uk/

Cherwell Scientific Publishing Ltd
The Magdalen Centre
Oxford Science Park
Oxford OX4 4GA
UK
Tel: +44 (0)1865 784800
Fax: +44 (0)1865 784801
E-mail: info@cherwell.com
Web Site: http://www.cherwell.com/

Biosoft
37 Cambridge Place
Cambridge CB2 1NS
UK
Tel : +44 (0)1223-368622
Fax : +44 (0)1223-312873
E-mail: info@biosoft.com
Web Site: http://www.biosoft.com/biosoft/

Research Information Systems Inc
Bilaney Consultants Ltd
St Julians
Sevenoaks
Kent TN15 0RX
UK
Tel : +44 (0)1732-450002
Fax : +44 (0)1732-450003
E-mail: bilaney@bilaney.com
Web Site: http://www.bilaney.com/

Smart Software
40 Castle Ings Gardens
Leeds
LS12 5EG
Tel : +44 (0)113-263-1388
E-mail: sales@smart-software.com
Web Site: http://www.smart-software.com

ENVOI

'Until more is known about what works and why practitioners change practice, all NHS facilities and the Department of Health should exhibit large signs saying:

In God we trust. All others bring data.'

Prof Alan Maynard
Guardian
17 July 1996

Index